# Double Pregnant

# Double Pregnant

Natalie Meisner

Two Lesbians Make a Family

**Roseway Publishing**
an imprint of Fernwood Publishing
Halifax & Winnipeg

*A Note on Potential Donors*: I wrote about our journey with candor and humour, but I believe in the Hippocratic Oath for writers as well as for doctors: First, do no harm. And so in cases where I thought the potential donor could be "outed" or exposed by what I wrote, I protected them by making changes to their geographical location, occupation or other identifying factors.

Editing and text design: Brenda Conroy
Cover artwork: Painting "Double Pregnant" by Laurence Hämmerli
Cover design: John van der Woude
Printed and bound in Canada

Published by Roseway Publishing
an imprint of Fernwood Publishing
32 Oceanvista Lane, Black Point, Nova Scotia, B0J 1B0
and 748 Broadway Avenue, Winnipeg, Manitoba, R3G 0X3
www.fernwoodpublishing.ca/roseway

Fernwood Publishing Company Limited gratefully acknowledges the financial support of the Government of Canada through the Canada Book Fund, the Canada Council for the Arts, the Nova Scotia Department of Tourism and Culture and the Province of Manitoba, through the Book Publishing Tax Credit, for our publishing program.

   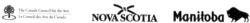 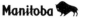

Library and Archives Canada Cataloguing in Publication

Meisner, Natalie D., 1972-, author
Double pregnant : two lesbians make a family / Natalie Meisner.

ISBN 978-1-55266-601-2 (pbk.)

1. Meisner, Natalie D., 1972- --Family. 2. Lesbian couples--Biography. 3. Pregnancy. 4. Lesbianism. I. Title.

HQ75.4.M45A3 2014      306.76'63092      C2013-908696-X

*To my beloved wife, Viviën,*
*whose grand idea all of this was*

# Contents

1. tea for two  /  1

2. flat out no  /  4

3. the kindness of strangers  /  7

4. speed dating for sperm donors  /  10

5. under construction  /  13

6. the arbiter of my own suffering  /  15

7. put mommy down  /  19

8. queerer than we can suppose  /  21

9. I know how to swim  /  22

10. those Nobelists could never win a basketball game  /  27

11. why wasn't I born a lesbian  /  30

12. elevation is important  /  33

13. Indomitable Lions  /  38

14. (still) under construction  /  41

15. busted flat in Banff  /  42

16. house call  /  50

17. the weight of each breast  /  55

18. eighty percent pregnant  /  56

19. out damn spot  /  58

20. endgame  /  59

21. there's the rub  /  65

22. better than no sperm at all  /  68

23. bigdaddybear  /  71

24. contemplating anonymity  /  76

25. leaning dangerously from a fourth-storey
      window in Vienna  /  81

26. hitchhiker to the candy store  /  83

27. separating the nuts  /  85

28. make the call  /  88

29. a walk in the park  /  89

30. *to the Sylvia on rollerblades* / 90

31. *letters to possible creatures (dear baby to be)* / 94

32. *out of the blue* / 95

33. *pluses and minuses* / 96

34. *X's and O's* / 97

35. *dykes and tykes on bikes* / 97

36. *partnering with the floor* / 98

37. *letters to possible creatures (kwispelen)* / 103

38. *maximum fecundity or Escher stymied* / 104

39. *womb with a view* / 105

40. *ad nauseum* / 107

41. *letters to possible creatures (dear tadpole)* / 107

42. *bumper sticker logic* / 109

43. *Wilson* / 110

44. *trying again in Peachland with a separated rib* / 111

45. *lucky* / 114

46. *Pachelbel or Hendrix?* / 117

47. *training for it* / 119

48. *control is a thing you learn to lose* / 120

49. *fear itself* / 122

50. *crossing the bridge* / 125

51. *smallmedium@large* / 128

52. *sublime bean* / 130

53. *why do they call it morning sickness* / 132

54. *boy business* / 132

55. *oxytocin cocktail* / 135

56. *call the networks* / 136

57. *letters to possible creatures (on how you came to be)* / 138

58. *the belly says no* / 139

59. *the old wives say* / 139

60. *the sweetest drumbeat in the world* / 140

61. *measuring up like a twenty-year-old* / 142

62. *gayby boom* / 144

63. *jaws of life* / 146

64. *stay put till we get back to the ocean* / 147

65. *cosmic weights and balances* / 148

66. *should old acquaintance be forgot* / 149

67. *a prayer upon leaving* / 150

68. *mamaburger* / 153

69. *not Hollywood* / 156

70. *nipple stimulation, spicy food & pineapples* / 158

71. *from a distance, a penguin* / 161

72. *letters to possible creatures (on people I wish
        you'd known)* / 162

73. *following survivor* / 163

74. *we have created enchantment* / 164

75. *sleep of the righteously exhausted* / 168

76. *unlearning* / 170

77. *of zen & concrete* / 171

78. *on the monitor* / 172

79. *a new project* / 179

*Acknowledgements* / 181

## 1. tea for two

My wife and I are out on the dance floor in a downtown bar in Calgary, when she pops the question. The music pulses with a syncopated bass beat — *oonch, oonch, oonch* — and dancers bob and weave around us on all sides while lasers shower the floor, the wall and our bodies. Outside, snow is howling around the streetlamps and drifting up over the hoods of the cars. We have ventured out into a mad January blizzard, the kind of storm that would bring things to a grinding halt nearly anywhere else in the world but out here on the Canadian prairie only makes people seriously commit to snow tires.

We have gone out in this blizzard to avoid cabin fever. To put a finer point on it, I have dragged my wife, Viviën, out into this weapons grade winter storm because I am afraid that she is going to get cabin fever and then leave me.

You see, Viviën moved to Canada so we could be together. She grew up in Holland, but when I met her she had already relocated to the sunny South of France because she found the Netherlands too cold and wet. Shock and awe would best describe the look on her face the first time she walked out into a true sub-forty Alberta clipper. Whenever the temperature dips below minus ten I start to watch for luggage in the hallway. Someone who moved here from the Midi-Pyrénées, after all, is pretty much impervious to the sturdy prairie assurance that it might be cold, yes, *but it's a dry cold.*

I am floored by what I think she's just said, and so I freeze, stop dancing mid-beat and yell: "What?" She cups my elbows in her palms and I look up into her eyes.

"Do you want to have a baby with me?" She asks, and my world tilts sideways on its axis. I am just a little bit tipsy so the force of the question itself is enough to cause me to stumble backward a bit. She steadies me and tilts me upright.

*Do you want to have a baby with me?* Now there is a question that can sweep you off your feet.

As a tomboy in rural Nova Scotia one of my main objectives growing up was to get out of town *without* having a baby. I saw so many of my friends having children while they, themselves, were barely grown, and I knew I wanted to see the world. It seemed enough to hope to get out unscathed — that I could escape and create a life filled with books, with learning, with travel, was beyond imagining. Also, at a fairly early age I realized that I might love women. At that time, of course, there was no such thing as gay marriage. In fact, in a small town such as ours, it was barely acknowledged that there were gay *people*.

How, then, could I ever have dreamt that one day I would meet a woman from halfway around the world and fall in love? That I would be able to walk with her hand-in-hand down the street? That colleagues and family members alike from far and wide would not only tolerate our relationship (tolerance being of very little worth in a pinch) but accept it with the respect and honour they give their own? That I would one day get down on one knee, just like I had seen in the movies, and ask the one I love to marry me? Lastly, how could I ever have dared to dream that my beloved would be standing in front of me, out on the dance floor, asking me this question, but here we are.

Now would be a good time to let you know how much I love kids. Babies in the strollers of strangers passing by reach out their arms for me. Toddlers in restaurants identify me as the one most willing to spend the rest of dinner playing funny face ping-pong. In my very large extended family (one grandmother had thirteen children, the other had six), I've always been happy with the role of favourite cousin/auntie who's never too tired to play. Kayak, fish, surf in the chilly Atlantic, hunt frogs, you name it, they know I'm game. I never get tired of their questions and actually pepper them with my own for fun. But a family of my own? A baby? Or babies of our own to feed, clothe, burp, love and care for every single day until they are full grown? I never thought about it, I guess because I thought it was out of reach for me.

Here is a major fork in the road. After I answer this question, I will no longer be the same person I was before it was posed. This is the question I never dared ask myself. This is the question — suddenly this feeling washes over me like a big bottle-green breaker in the Atlantic — that I have been waiting for. Viviën has picked the lock of the innermost chamber of my heart with a few simple words, and the answer is written there, etched plainly on the wall: *I do*. It says. *Especially with you.*

Around us the music plays on. The DJ is infusing a Motown classic with a Bollywood hit … *Mama said, you can't hurry love, no you just have to wait* … the sitar and the tabla kick in, layered in over drum and bass, and the dancers dig it, shaking their hips and waving fists in the air. *She said love don't come easy, now it's a game of give and take.*

They've turned on the black light. Teeth and eyes light up, incandescent. Young men in a lather of sweat peel off their shirts and twirl them overhead like towels at a soccer match. A sharp crack — balls scatter as pool-playing lesbians angle around the table contemplating their shot while keeping one eye on the entrance. An athletic girl with short shaggy hair and a nose ring drapes her arm sweetly, drunkenly, around a girl she is chatting up. Next to me someone shakes her beer and sprays a friend who squeals and jumps back. Some of the beer splashes me and the shaker flashes me a sheepish smile and mouths "sorry" over the music. At the pool table another girl flashes her breasts quickly to distract the shooter. It is a lively good time on a Saturday night and we stand in the middle of it all, frozen to the spot in wonder, until one of our friends comes over and smacks me on the shoulder.

"You two look really cute together, but you need to get a room!" She makes the "call me" sign and then is gone.

Viviën and I begin to make heady plans for the future. *Why stop at one baby, let's have two!* We don't notice the patrons gradually leaving in ones and twos to brave the storm. We don't notice the music stopping, the staff cleaning up or the lights coming on.

Finally a handsome young bartender comes over to us. He is drying up the last beer glass. "Okay ladies," he says. "I'm going home now. You want me to leave you the keys and you can lock up?" We laugh, shrug our jackets outside and are hit with a wall of light fluffy snow. The wind has stopped and the snow floats gently down. We hold hands in our mittens and struggle through the drifts. It is so still that our questions seem to hang in the soft winter air as if suspended in cartoon speech balloons. *Who will carry the baby? One of us? Maybe we should both try? Maybe we can have two and that way they'll be siblings? Do we care if we have a boy or a girl?*

It doesn't really matter, but one of each would be great and I sing, badly ... *Tea for two, and two for tea. Me for you and you for me. We can raise a fam-i-ly, a boy for you and a girl for me...*

## 2. flat out no

Deciding that we want to raise children together gives us such a rush that we float around on fluffy clouds of possibility for a few days. *How will it feel to cup their tiny heels in the palms of our hand? What about their first step? Their first word?* It is a heady period as we prepare for our lives to change. After a week or two things get complicated. Bringing children into the world isn't a simple prospect even for a straight/fertile couple, but for us, a lesbian couple in our thirties, one quite practical impediment to pregnancy emerged immediately: We can't just go off the pill and wait for nature to take its course.

So we begin trying out different scenarios of how we might get ourselves knocked up. We sift through our male friends and acquaintances for possible donors. We talk briefly about adoption, but Viviën does not want to adopt. She, herself was adopted. She is a black woman of Suriname/Dutch descent who was adopted into a white family. She only found out the identity of her biological mother and father when she was a teenager. Her feelings about biology and attachment are shaped, of course, by her experience; they are strong and they are particular. She wants a biological connection to the children. She also wants them to be related by blood to one another if at all possible. I am less concerned with blood relations, but that is perhaps because I am not adopted, and so we have to honour her feelings on this aspect.

Given these strong preferences, you might think the logical choice for us would be to head for the local sperm bank, choose an anonymous donor and purchase some samples. That, however, is also a problem for her. Despite a happy and peaceful childhood with her adoptive parents and brother, Viviën tells me that the question of her biological parents weighed on her throughout her young life. For this reason, it's very important to her that our children be able to get in touch with their biological father if they want to. Even if it is only later in their lives. Most clinics deal solely with anonymous donors. This means that the identities of both the sperm donor and recipient are protected. Only one clinic in Canada offers an open identity option. We could choose a donor who has ticked off the open ID box, but that tick is not binding. So even though we might tell any resulting children that they have the right, when they turn eighteen, to learn the identity of their biological father, the donor might have changed his mind, and that would be that.

I understand a clinic's caution. The intent is to protect the donor who never wanted parental responsibilities in the first place from having them thrust upon him. However, this does make it more difficult to honour Viviën's strong preference. And then again we have other misgivings about sperm clinics. We think it's unfair that gay men aren't allowed to be donors. As well, we find it impersonal and alienating to be flipping through a catalogue and shopping for a dad for our baby.

We have discussions late into the night about how we can best navigate these uncharted waters. On the one hand our discussions are practical: *What friend can we turn to for a favour such as this?* And dreamy on the other hand: *We'll teach them three languages, they'll have two passports and the world will be their international oyster.* We picture ourselves courtside at all their games. As basketball players ourselves, we take it as an article of faith that our children will want to play too. *We'll try to open the world up for them but also allow them to make their own mistakes. We'll teach them the value of hard work, of kindness, and the importance of the social contract.*

Plans and dreams such as these consume us through the fluffy snow days and the vicious winds of a prairie winter. Finally it dawns on us that no amount of inspired conversation will cause a baby to materialize out of the ether. We'll have to leap that frightening chasm between talk and action. We can wax poetic about sunny days in the park and sandcastles on the shoreline; we can visualize their first steps and pick out our favourite books to read to them. We can imagine saying to them in the quasi-distant future: *Finished your homework? Good, now go get Mommy a beer so she can kick your ass at pool.* We can rehearse child-rearing techniques till the cows come home … but if we really want a family, we are going to need some help. We are going to have to get down to brass tacks. I'll say it plain: We are going to need sperm. Lots of safe fresh sperm with high motility rates. And a fellow willing to give it to us with very few strings attached.

My first thought is to ask an old friend. He is a writer and traveller that I've known since undergraduate days at Dalhousie University. We were in a poetry class studying Shelley's "Ode to the West Wind" when we got to the line: *I fall upon the thorns of life! I bleed!*

The professor asked, "Has anyone here fallen upon the thorns of life?"

My friend says he noticed me for the first time when I was the only one in a lecture hall of a hundred and fifty people to put up my hand. Funny how memory works; I remember him raising his hand. Nonetheless we became fast friends — writing, reading each other's drafts, swapping books, arguing and talking into the wee hours of frosty Halifax mornings. It was with him that I shared many of those earnest pitchers of beer that foster conversations you are sure can change the world.

He's the perfect donor. He's intelligent, accomplished, open-minded and very funny. I imagine him filling a rather heroic and not too taxing spot in our extended family. I even have a chic twenty-first-century handle picked out for him. We can call him the *biodad*. After the initial spot of help, he can skip over the all the messy inconvenient stages that babies pass through, where liquids leak out of one end and noises issue from the other, and just be there for the fun parts.

My friend had never indicated that he wanted children of his own. In fact he had always scorned ties of any sort so I imagine that this could be a boon to him. *What time zone is the biodad in right now?* We'll ask the children when they're learning to tell time. *Want to Skype him and show him your volcano project?* Or he can pop by for a visit on a layover from New York to Bangkok. We'll have the babies all washed and applecheeked, well fed and cheerful. He can bounce the little ones on his knee and bask in the glow of having done a really good thing while we cook him an excellent meal. After the kids are in bed we can sit around the fire while he regales us with exciting tales of his life in the global trenches while we supply heartwarming anecdotes of family life.

We can live vicariously through one another over rounds of single malt. It was such an elaborate fantasy that I realize I must have been unconsciously shading in the details for some time.

But my old friend rocks me with a serious mental uppercut when he says no. I don't mean, "Not right now, let me think about it." Not "I'm honoured, but…" I mean he flat out rejects me. He provides a rationale for the decision and it runs roughly along these lines: The world is a mess, he doesn't want to bring a child onto a planet that is hedonistically hurtling toward self destruction … and he had just read Cormac McCarthy's *The Road*. This particular dystopian novel does leave a lasting impression. So strong, apparently, that my friend equates giving us sperm to winding up the lone sane survivor on a lifeless, sunless planet where he alone must defend our progeny from legions of cannibalistic lunatics.

This isn't quite the future that I had in mind when I pitched the idea to him, and I'd like to say I am *disappointed*. Because it sounds so much more grown up. But closer to the truth, I am pissed. And hurt. My thinking runs something like this:

*Seriously? This is something you could do in five minutes — give or take, I'm a little rusty in this department — which could change the whole course of our lives. How can you just flat out refuse me?*

Of course I know it might be complicated. He would have to talk about this with his girlfriend, whom I haven't yet met, and see what her feelings are on the subject. The logistics could also prove challenging. He doesn't live in Calgary and his job takes him all over the world. My friend teaches English as a second language and goes wherever the money is good. He changes continents like he changes his socks. But I thought we could figure all of this out with some good will and creative flight bookings. I wanted to offer him some of the fringe benefits of fatherhood and none of the horrible green poop.

I had thought of every single aspect of how great it would be if he were our donor. I had not, not even for a second, looked into the future to think about how I would feel if he said no. I hadn't anticipated the bizarre sense of rejection that came with his no. I guess that I also hadn't stopped to think about things from his point of view. Of course contributing his genetic material would complicate his life in a profound way. The symbolic weight of having a being out there in the world with half of your biological information would be powerful. It is powerful, there is no denying it. Otherwise why would *we* be putting so much thought into exactly the same thing?

Aha moment. Too bad I didn't have it then. If I'd had it then, I might not have felt like the only strike-out at some bizarre reproductive Sadie Hawkins dance.

## 3. the kindness of strangers

After the first rejection, we are a bit gun-shy of asking any other friends to help us out. I have to actively stop myself from cruising every new and interesting man I meet as a potential donor. We often wish that we each had a relative we could ask to be a donor for the other as this is a path many lesbian couples take in order to keep those familial connections.

For my part, I had a younger cousin I was very close to that I might have asked this favour of. When he died recently at the age of twenty-three, it was me who gave his eulogy. The task of summing up a life like his — so promising yet hacked off at the root — is a thankless one. It's been a couple of years now since his death, and the missing of him now grabs me only when I am alone. My chest will tighten when I am at a stoplight on my way home from work and I'll remember him at different ages: four years old, lying on his back on spring green grass eating cherries; fourteen, getting that teenager skulk but still a hint of a smile for me; or twenty-one, with his cobra tattoo right after his first overdose. It is a sad story and one I don't have the heart to tell here in full. I miss him a lot. I am an only child and he was as close to a brother as I'll ever have. The fact that he would have been the one I was most comfortable turning to for a favour like this only makes the missing of him worse.

"What about your brother?" I ask Viviën as we sit down for our by-now-familiar evening glass of wine/baby-making brainstorm session. I met him several times on our visits to Holland and like him very much. "That is as close as we can come to having a baby related to both of us."

She nods and, a testament to her time living in France, considers this while giving a cute little sniff at the rim of the glass before sipping. So hard to get good wine here. Another strike against frigid Canada.

I go on. "Yes! You two have so many traits in common. He's smart and funny and strong. He has your eyes. And he's really cute, too."

"*Gek*," she says, which means "crazy" in Dutch. "This is getting weird."

"You know, for a boy," I reply.

"But that means that if we both have a baby, they can never be related."

"True. Which we want," I agree.

"Yes. It's important for them," she confirms.

There is also the question of actually making the ask. As we now know, being turned down stirs up a whole nest of emotions. That person you ask to give you their ejaculate will never be able to look at you in exactly the same way again, despite everyone's best intentions. The stakes are so high that there is probably no way to ask this question of a close friend or relative that doesn't risk some fall-out to the relationship unless the outcome is positive.

Shortly after this conversation, Viviën gets news from her brother that puts this line of thinking to rest. Her brother and his wife are expecting their own baby, and we are overjoyed for them. It feels like a violation of some unwritten rule if we were to ask him to be our donor now. When happiness strikes loved ones it is important to be able to simply share it with them, purely, untouched by the blueprints of your own plans and dreams.

I had, however, already begun to picture this little son or daughter that we might have conceived with her brother, and so when we close this door I can't help but feel a pang. A marked and distinct sadness as if I am saying goodbye. Goodbye to a prospect. Goodbye before even a hello. I can now feel the rhythm of something like a metronome begin to swing through me. A kind of steady beat somewhere deep in my gut that keeps insisting on a baby. Is it a ticking?

*Tick-tock, tick tock.* The biological clock that is supposed to be wound up like some kind of time bomb and ticking away inside each and every woman's blessed womb. *Essentialist sexist claptrap!* I thought and still do. And yet … I seem to have suddenly sprouted one of these clocks. Either that or I have swallowed Captain Hook's crocodile with his arm and an alarm clock inside.

It hits me suddenly: *I'm afraid.*

We really want this. We really want to raise a family together. What if it proves impossible?

To let yourself want something. No … someone. To *really* want someone … leaves you absolutely no idea of how to keep going with your life if they are not in it, and it is terrifying. It's like admitting you are in love without knowing if you're loved in return.

This is the moment I start communicating with little beings who don't yet exist. I whisper tiny wishes to the air, the sky, to my own belly and to Viviën's.

*I want you.* I say to the baby who could take root inside her. *You are welcome.* I murmur to these beings who could jump on us, squealing with delight, and wake us up on lazy Sunday mornings of the future.

Even, *I need you.* With no stop-gaps, no contingencies and no back-up plan. No way to make this okay if you decide not to arrive.

Prevailing upon a family member to be our donor isn't an option. I asked a friend and it didn't work out. I briefly consider asking my boss. He and his partner are forward thinking individuals, great conversationalists and know how to throw a dinner party. But again, what if he says no? Those hallway chats could become squirmy affairs for both of us. Most of Viviën's close male friends are all the way across the Atlantic in Holland. If we really want this to happen we are going to have to get creative. We are going to have to look for someone who will see this as an opportunity. Someone who is neither shy about biological matters nor precious about his genetic material. And lastly someone who we do not yet know.

Tennessee Williams' *A Streetcar Named Desire* is on my syllabus this term. As I re-read it in preparation for class, the plight of Blanche Dubois strikes me closer to the heart than ever before. Viviën and I both use power tools and drive pick-up trucks. Viviën is an engineer, has a pilot's licence for small aircraft and does some welding on the side. We are about as far from the southern belle as two women can be ... and yet here we are: we have arrived at a place in our lives where we are about to rely upon the kindness of strangers. I am not sure, however, that we live in a world where you can depend upon a stranger for anything, let alone a favour so intimate and so important.

## 4. speed dating for sperm donors

So where do you turn when you need to find a likely stranger? Why, to that vast repository of human knowledge, that colossal ocean of red herrings called the internet. After hours of research, with extra time to play "Wac-a-Mole" with the porn pop-ups that fly toward me when I type in "sperm donor" on the search engine, I find some legitimate sites for people who are in the same boat as we are.

The boat is called the SS *Infertility* and I'm surprised to find it crowded with people from all walks of life. From first class to steerage, all of us trying to gain the peaceful harbour of family life. Viviën and I look at site after site where women, gay and straight, married and single, pour their hearts out on the topic of conception. It is frightening to realize just how many obstacles from the biological to the financial to the social there are to conceiving a child. On the other hand, our searches provide some comfort. You can't help but feel a sense of kinship to all those other women out there with a similar hunger in their bellies.

Some sites take a cheerful approach with names like DIY Baby. This site focuses on practical advice for the first-time self-inseminator. Based in the U.K., DIY Baby makes getting yourself or your wife pregnant with donor sperm seem as simple as throwing up a sheet of drywall in the basement or fixing a leaky faucet.

A site called Co-parent.net offers a whole spectrum of new and intriguing models for a family. There are single men and women looking to find someone with whom they can have and raise a child, but without a romantic relationship. There are gay couples and single gay men looking for either light involvement or full-on co-parenting arrangements with women. There are gay men looking for surrogates with an open adoption clause. Single women who want to parent alone. In short, there are individuals and couples of nearly every walk of life, gender and identity affiliation all looking for some version of the same thing: continuity. A family. A way to love, to pass something on, to pay it forward I suppose.

Still other sites, like FSDW (Free Sperm Donations Worldwide), act as a hub for potential donors and recipients to connect. There we find an astonishing number of men from all over the world offering their services as donors. Some men are willing to travel to you, if you pay their airfare and expenses. Others offer to ship their sperm via FedEx. Some men post pictures of themselves, even of children they have fathered. The pictures make me squirm. These children could hardly consent to having their pictures posted as a kind of unorthodox résumé.

There are a couple of important abbreviations that anyone entering this brave new world needs to add to their vocabulary. AI and NI stand for artificial and natural insemination, respectively. Some men have a strict preference for one or the other. Not surprisingly, Viviën and I are all about the AI option.

After familiarizing ourselves with the new jargon and the protocol, we begin to talk about how we will write an ad of our own. Since I am the writer, the actual drafting falls to me. My first attempt at a tag line looks like this: *Professional Lesbian Couple Seeking Donor.*

We hold it at arm's length and inspect.

"That makes it seem like we're getting paid," says Viviën.

"What?"

"The words professional and lesbian together," she laughs.

"Ah. I see the problem. Like we went pro. Hey, that's not a bad idea. Maybe we could get some sponsorships. Hello, Nike? Converse? "

We take a few more runs at it together. It is actually quite a difficult piece of text to compose. You want to cast a wide net ... but not too wide. You want to sound approachable ... but not desperate. You want to give some men a reason to write to you ... but you don't want to come off like you're flogging a set of encyclopaedia. After scratching our heads and drafting out loud we come up with the following:

> *Hi! We are a married couple (two women) looking for a sperm donor to help us start a family. We are not looking for a co-parent, but are open to the possibility of a donor being a part of the child's life.*
>
> *A bit about us: we are a writer and an engineer hailing from Nova Scotia and Holland, respectively. We work on renovation projects in our spare time, play basketball and soccer and enjoy the outdoors. We are sociable, easy going and like to travel and have dinner parties. If you are interested please contact us to discuss further.*

I am not sure, at this point, where we sit on the easy-going scale, but I have faith that we can be, again, once we manage to get ourselves pregnant. The site doesn't require it, but most people have chosen to, so we even post a photo of us crouching down on a pier with water and mountains in the background. Our intrepid pup (a blue heeler Aussie mix) sits there with us, perking up his ears for the picture.

The site has its own email system, and we begin getting messages almost immediately, which is very exciting. Our first message is from an enthusiastic and horny twenty-two-year-old going by the name of Delbert.

"Hey, look, we got our first message," I call out to Viviën, who is stirring a pot of something fragrant in the kitchen. I catch wafts of cinnamon ... cardamom. Maybe her trademark lamb stock/squash soup?

"And there are pictures. Lots of shirtless pictures."

"What? What does he say?"

"He says he can drive down here immediately from Edmonton ... at least he's close by ... and get this: take as much time as needed to get as many women pregnant as we like."

"How many women does he think we have over here?"

"Well the ad says two," I say.

Viviën comes running over, ladle in hand, leaving a trail of soup drops across the kitchen floor. "But we said AI. We said artificial insemination. *As needed*? He did not say that!"

"Read it yourself. There's no way I could make that up." And there isn't. This is only the first in a series of events that take us into *terra incognita* and put us into situations far stranger than fiction.

## 5. *under construction*

Viviën and I have a house that sits at the mouth of the harbour in the Nova Scotian fishing village of about five hundred people called Lockeport. Today you'll see a well cared for salt-cured Cape Cod with silvery wooden siding, a cozy outdoor fire pit and a little writing cabin/ guest space at the water's edge. However, the house wasn't really a house when I bought it nine years ago,. It had been uninhabited for some time. The roofline was starting to give, the old stacked stone foundation had slid, and the walls needed work. It was more like an idea of a house — a dream of a house that once was and could be again.

I grew up nearby with many of my relatives either fishing or making their livelihood in some other way from the sea. Even though work and personal life have taken me far away from the Atlantic for nearly twenty years (Montreal, Yellowknife, Vancouver, Connecticut, Regina and now Calgary), some part of me still feels the tide ebbing and flowing each day on the beaches and shorelines I roamed as a child.

Moving around this much can produce an intense craving for a place to think of as home. When I first stood on the steps of the old house, I detected bits of green paint that had blistered and peeled, leaving only the weathered wood underneath. The wind whipped around the corners of the house, and I spied the simple piece of painted boat board with a screw through that served as a lock. I turned it, opened the door and went up the stairs. As I stepped inside, the house breathed the word "home" into my ear, and so when I got my first full-time teaching position

I bought it. I bought it knowing I would always have to be someplace else for work. I bought it with no idea how or when I'd be able to fix it. I bought it strictly for the feeling of home that it gave me and that I badly needed. Thus I become either the town's laughing stock or the Patron Saint of Old Houses, depending on who you ask.

The house had no plumbing, no electricity, ancient lathes and plaster on the walls and only eelgrass stuffed inside the walls for insulation. What it lacked in comfort and amenities, however, it made up for in soul. It was one of the first homesteads erected when the town was settled as Locke's Island. It housed generations of fishermen and fishermen's sons and daughters, and their stories are practically worn right into the grain of the wide floorboards, worn velvety smooth, not by machines but by the passage of so many feet. The house belonged to the much beloved Celia, or Celie Turner as local people call her, a descendant of one of Lockeport's original Black Loyalist families. I bought it from her niece, Marjorie Turner-Bailey, the accomplished sprinter who represented Canada in the 1976 Olympics. All during our renovation process Marjorie stops by to see how the work is coming, often bringing a gift of mussels or clams that she has gathered for us herself.

Though the house is not large, Celie had taken advantage of the prime location near the wharf and built a number of bunk rooms, which she rented out to fishermen. All along one wall were hooks where their gear would have hung and markings in the wood where the salt water dripped off. Long after I'd purchased the house, I learned from a book called *The Lost Mariners of Shelburne County* that my own grandfather (just arrived from Newfoundland) and grandmother met at a party in this very house. One of my uncles later lived in Celie's bunk house, and I found a swordfish he had carved hanging on the back of one of the doors.

To this day, when we sit on the back steps, which are actually right in the middle of the road that leads to the wharf, people stop and share a memory about Celie: *She gave me a whole haddock one day*, or *I ran to the store for her five days out of the week*. It is likely that the house will forever be called Celie's house, and that is fine with us.

Before Viviën and I met, I had been trying each summer, with the help of relatives and the expertise of local workmen, to accomplish some of the major structural repairs. The first year we jacked up the house, replaced the huge sills (the large pieces of wood that run the length of the house and hold it up) and poured a new concrete foundation. The following year came new windows and doors, and the year after that, new long-board wooden siding. Bit by bit the elegant little house squared her shoulders and shored up against the elements. The outside of the house returned to her former dignity. Of course, if you actually wanted to live there, all this work was quite beside the point. There was still no electricity, plumbing or interior to speak of.

Viviën and I had decided that this summer we would do a total reconstruction of the interior of Celie's house. Viviën is an engineer by trade and had done restorations on an old stone farm house in France and several apartments in Holland. She drew up a floor plans and we resolved to work in a small team, composed of us two, one of my cousins and two travelling workers from the U.K. who wanted to spend some time in Nova Scotia.

With so much physical construction underway (not to mention the futility of trying to find a sperm donor in a town of 500, fully half of whom are my cousins), we decide to put our baby-making project on hold until we return to Calgary in September. We continue communicating with potential donors over the summer, hoping to find the right match for our return. We pound, hammer, saw, mud and paint until the inside of the house begins to look more and more like a home. Each evening, tired and covered with a light frosting of sawdust, we sit down and write to potential donors or hatch plans and schemes to make our little family bigger.

## 6. the arbiter of my own suffering

In addition to websites, we also put the word out through local networks and friends in the west to let them know that we are looking for a donor. It is in this way that we meet a gay couple from Vancouver with whom we seem to have a lot in common. They like to travel and cook, so do we. They are active in local sports organizations … hey, we love sports. They are part of the local arts and culture scene… and the list goes on.

We exchanged a few emails over the summer and it turned out they would be visiting Calgary in September for business. One of them is a foodie and so he chooses a restaurant for us all to meet and get acquainted. Meeting them outside a funky tapas restaurant on Stephen Avenue, we are a bit surprised to find that neither of them, even to the tops of their perfectly coifed faux-hawks, stands as high as Viviën's breasts. As we are introducing ourselves in a four-square formation, I can feel them craning their necks to look up at Viviën, and I register her own surprise as she looks down.

Height alone is no reason to count them out. There's no call to go discriminating against the less-tall of the world. And besides, height isn't always passed down biologically, is it? And even if it is, so what? Have we let our overactive imaginations about our future daughter or son the basketball star run away with us? Are we height bigots? I already feel that a wholesale interrogation of my heretofore unexamined prejudice against the vertically challenged is in order when suddenly I am rescued.

These two cannot be our donors, it becomes clear before the appetizers arrive, and it has nothing to do with their height. It isn't their shortness that disqualifies this couple. No, it is the foodie blogger treatise we are bludgeoned with on the art of the vinaigrette before the menus come. It is the rehearsal of each and every entry for each and every restaurant the slightly taller one wrote in the past six months. The excoriation he gave the Italian restaurant for serving herb-infused bread. The wrath he has for the new French place on Fourth that served something *they call* a pissaladière when it was clearly a tourtière. And on and on.

Some people didn't take kindly to what he wrote about their establishment on his blog, he lets us know, and he has no idea why that could be unless it is because they are unwashed, uneducated, uncouth savages. We wonder how we might survive future coffee dates or dinner parties with these would-be biodaddies. There is nothing like an exacting foodie to just plain suck all the fun out of a good dinner. And indeed the process of deciding upon which dishes we will order at the lovely little tapas restaurant involves so much prevarication, so many false starts and so much sniper fire between the two men that Viviën and I begin to eyebrow each other. *Whose idea was this,* her eyebrows ask me.

*Mine. But what other options do we have?* Mine reply, chagrined.

The couple across from us, now apparently convinced that we know one another well enough, drop the kid gloves and begin to fight in earnest. People in the restaurant take sidelong glances toward our table. The slightly taller one berates the slightly shorter one about his choices. We, apparently, aren't allowed to order anything at all.

Viviën catches the waiter's attention when Slightly Taller isn't looking. "Braised riblets," she whispers behind her hand. Tones escalate. Dirty looks are exchanged. Are they on their best behaviour, I can't help wondering. Why don't they want to make a better impression on us? Viviën and I hold hands under the table while a verbal tennis match ensues.

"I *want* the miso-encrusted halibut bites," Slightly Shorter says.

"You ordered them last time and they were greasy," replies Slightly Taller.

We shift in our seats. I begin to feel that the chairs are hard. So hard that my ass desperately wants to go home to the sofa.

"You never let me order," says Slightly Shorter .

"I do. Lord only knows how many greasy halibut bites I've choked down at your behest."

"Culinary martyrs of the world, we salute you," and Slightly Shorter mock claps for emphasis.

"Puhleez don't let this be a repeat of Tampa," warns Slightly Taller.

That is puzzling, and I wonder for a moment if I might drop in an interrogative … Tampa? To see if I could flip the switch on the line and reroute this train wreck of a dinner.

Slightly Shorter: "I never get anything I want."

Slightly Taller: "You got to have the wedding Stateside, where all *your* friends could make it."

Slightly Shorter: "That's only because if we had it here, you don't have any friends, and wouldn't that be embarrassing."

Slightly Shorter is beginning to reach the end of his rope. He is fighting back. Slightly Taller rolls up his sleeves and decides not to bite on that hook. Instead he returns to the menu scrum.

Slightly Taller: "Not only were they greasy, the bites, they were limp."

Slightly Shorter: "That won't be the only encounter with limpness I'll have this evening, I'll wager."

The waiter finally comes with the dish that Viviën ordered. Slightly Taller waves it off summarily, and Viviën has to rescue it as the waiter comes around the other side of the table.

"Actually I do want that," Viviën ventures and Slightly Taller pinions her with his eyes but she does not back down.

"I did order it, and I do want to eat it," Viviën, having had enough, pronounces evenly.

By the time the desert cards arrive, Viviën and I are dissolving into fits of suppressed hysterical giggles. We had tried asking direct questions about their work, hobbies, anything. But it only seemed to throw gas on the fire of whatever was simmering between them.

"The fact is," confides Slightly Taller, "he moved to the west coast from Toronto solely to be with me. He suffers from isolation and I pay the price."

"I think I should be the arbiter of my own suffering," Slightly Shorter states quietly, but Slightly Taller practises the art of selective hearing and continues. "He left behind everything, friends and family, the city he loves, to be with me. And so he deserves to be taken care of. He deserves the security that a full-time breadwinner gives him."

"Hm," I say, but I'm thinking: *Um, he's right here, he can hear you.*

Slightly Shorter eats his dame blanche with an emasculated and yet somehow ennobled look. He is taking the high road now, but dollars to doughnuts Slightly Taller will pay for this later.

By the time we get the cheque it occurs to me that Slightly Taller hasn't asked either of us one single question about what we think, what we do, why we might want to start a family, and in fact has displayed no curiosity whatsoever about the two potential vessels of his future progeny. Instead he has cut us off, ignored our attempts to enter the conversation, censored our dining choices (yet we do pay our half of the bill) and took constant shots at his husband. We simply couldn't imagine navigating all the necessary waters to reach the point of a donation with these two, never mind dealing with them for the next twenty years.

Finally, we all walk out onto the sidewalk. We are released into the cold Calgary night. The stars knife through the inky blackness, and I drink in the crisp air like a restorative tonic. The first breath of oxygen gives me some clarity after the stuffiness of the restaurant. Mostly because I don't know what to say and "call you later" sounds too cliché for words, I turn to Slightly Taller. Despite the fact that he has monopolized the conversation all evening with his foodie rhetoric, his blog, his family, his friends and despite the fact that he has spoken over the top of the rest of us, cut us off and generally just caterwauled without displaying the slightest flicker of interest in what kind of people the future mothers of the child he reputedly desires might be … I ask him, off the cuff, about his work.

"I am a corporate consultant in the field of communication," he says. "I study conversation. Actually it's quite fascinating…" And he is off. Yet another moment where truth just shoulders fiction aside and dashes over the finish line of life's race toward the bizarre.

## 7. put mommy down

Our next foray into strangerland in search of sperm proves even weirder. We are contacted by an ex-CFL linebacker who describes himself as six foot two, fit, smart and fun, with a great sense of humour. He adds that he is a card-carrying member of Mensa and a stanch Democrat who lives in San Diego and travels the world investing in oceanfront land, yachts and sports teams. I write to him that it might be difficult for him to be a donor for us since he lives in San Diego. No problem at all, he writes back. He can simply stop by Calgary on one of his intercontinental business trips. He sounds wonderful, and we wonder if it is reckless to invite a stranger — a stranger whose career included toppling 350-pound men, solid mountains of muscle, to the turf with his bare hands — into our home.

We are impressed that he would consider travelling all the way to Calgary to be our donor. He isn't looking to be a parent and he doesn't mind signing off on a donor agreement. He read our profile and thought we would make great mommies. He wants to help and hopes that maybe we could be friends afterward. His email nickname is Hulk, a name he says was given to him during his football days. Hulk, as in the Incredible Hulk. Viviën and I begin to imagine little green-hued toddlers, rippling muscles busting out of their onesies. They would rip up trees by the roots in the front yard. They would simply hoist us up over their heads when they don't want to come inside for naptime. *I mean it! Now! This is not funny. Put Mommy down!*

He strikes a casual tone in his emails and makes the whole process of giving us a fresh sperm donation seem simple and straightforward. And he seems like a great person. So great, in fact, that I start to have a bit of a tickle at the back of my skull. Why hasn't he sent the picture that he promised two emails ago? I ask for it again. He promises again to send a picture, but says he cannot at the moment as he is on his Blackberry and in Houston.

Neither of these factoids explain why he can't send a picture and we begin to wonder if he is indeed too good to be true — this independently wealthy, intellectual ex-linebacker. Emails with enthusiastic plans begin to proliferate in my inbox. He imagines us all hanging out, on the beach, having a clambake. *A clambake? This is a sperm donation not an Elvis movie.*

Still no photo arrives so we speculate that there is something drastically wrong with him. Does he have a third eye in the middle of his forehead? Is he a fourteen-year-old latch-key kid taking role-playing games to the next level?

Then messages start coming more frequently, and the tone bothers me in a way I can't quite put my finger on. Although we haven't yet met, he is becoming very familiar. Then, with no encouragement whatsoever from our end, he begins to compose scenes between the three of us using alarming idiom and faltering literary descriptors. "I can see the three of us chillaxin over a bottle of bubbly as the sun sets in the magenta sky," he writes. Now I can overlook the decidedly forced portmanteau, but I've spent the better part of my adult life around theatre people: I know the signs of full blown insanity when I read them.

Despite his email attachments showing he tested negative for every disease under the sun, his flurry of sperm motility reports (his sperm could run circles around any tight end in the CFL) and his general high spirits, we decide it is best to stop answering until he sends a photo.

When the photo does arrive, it is grainy and features him far in the background while two Bichon Frisés sit front and centre wearing vests and party hats, each lapping from its own tiny crystal bowl. Maybe I suffer from the lesbian prejudice against little dogs, but I feel that one Bichon Frisé on its own is objectionable. Having two and dressing them up should be an indictable offence. Viviën takes one look at the picture and cries "Next!" Now and then he still manages to nudge through my spam filter saying that he understands that he might not be the future biological father of our children, but he hopes we can still be friends.

## 8. queerer than we can suppose

I glance over at a book I am reading about genetics research. It is open to a black-and-white photo of J.B.S. Haldane, the early twentieth-century geneticist and biologist who, after his long and enthusiastic perusal of the natural world, made a wonderful distinction. Not only is the universe queerer than we suppose, he famously exclaimed, it is substantially queerer than we *can* suppose. Somehow, caught as we are in the middle of this our strange search, I find his words as comforting as a soft handmade quilt in a February nor'easter. The universe is *substantially* queerer than we can suppose. I stare at Haldane's photo.

What does his expression mean? Is that a wink or a squint? Or just the flat-out harassed curiosity of a rabid scientist chased by a hypothesis? The one eye that you can see is a positive laser beam of intelligence. What is the gesture? *Come hither? It's all in the details?* Is he pinching the tiny grain of sand upon which another limitless galaxy is perched? Is he saying A-OK ... or is he just on the edge of flipping us the bird? There is something of a ringmaster, of a PT Barnum in him. Look at that spit-slick part in his hair. Slap a sizing on that jawline. What a fabulous striped suit. What sartorial splendour! I find myself wondering if he would make a good sperm donor ... if he weren't long dead and a eugenics proponent to boot.

As we search for someone in the current historical moment to help us start a family, it seems like good idea to do some reading about the history of sperm donation. One quite spectacular incident points to some of the quandaries of paying for sperm. Joey Skaggs announced in 1975 that he was opening a celebrity sperm bank in Greenwich Village. He proposed to auction off samples from Mick Jagger, the Beatles (both the alive and dead ones), Bob Dylan, and even some very hip vintage sperm from Jimi Hendrix. On the morning the auction was to open, Skaggs and his lawyer announced it was a hoax. The fact that the celebrity sperm bank was a massive gag didn't stop women showing up in the hundreds wanting to buy sperm. Before it was widely acknowledged as a joke, the First Lady of American liberal feminism, Gloria Steinem, appeared on NBC to give the rock star sperm sale an award for bad taste. We could scoff at Steinem for failing to get the joke. We could also, with the benefit of hindsight, look down our noses at all those hopeful would-be moms lining up to buy non-existent rock star essence. Doesn't it serve them right for trying to reduce genius to biology? And even worse, to assign it a dollar value?

But I find myself unable to judge these women and their hopes and dreams. What were they looking for, after all? A little spark of talent or genius? A good back story for the child? What if a Dylan lyric had worked itself into the very fabric of their lives, the words becoming a kind of sacred earthly prayer? Isn't that in the same neighbourhood of what couples the world over hope for when they make a baby the old fashioned way? Blanche Dubois just won't leave me alone this year. She would empathize with the plight of the rock-star-sperm-buying would-be mothers. *I don't want realism,* she breathes, *I want magic! Yes, yes, magic. I do misrepresent things,* she admits when Stanley hog ties her with his thick rope of facts. *I don't tell truths. I tell what ought to be truth.*

## 9. I know how to swim

Our next potential donor is a lawyer. Not much else about him is revealed by his sparse profile but his geographical proximity is a good part of his appeal. Despite the last few disappointments, we've vowed to pursue every viable prospect. After all, we reason, you really can't tell who you'll be compatible with until you meet them in person. Also, there don't seem to be a legion of men in southern Alberta chomping at the bit to give an artificial sperm donation to a lesbian couple.

The fires of our urgency are stoked by the doctor we go to see at the fertility clinic. Peering over her funky Buddy Holly glasses and mincing no words, she breaks it down for us: "A woman's fertility begins to decline at twenty-seven, with a steep drop off at the age of thirty-five. At thirty-five you are considered of advanced maternal age. Your eggs are getting older by the day, so if you're serious about having a family you need to be aggressive."

It is frightening to think of any part of your body as having an expiration date. Maybe this is why we focus on the second part of her statement. We definitely want a family, so we will have to be aggressive. That appeals to the inner athlete in both of us. *Fast break! Let's go team! It's the bottom of the fourth quarter!*

Being aggressive means scrapping our orderly two-year plan. We had supposed that we would find a donor, get Viviën pregnant, have a baby, and then start the process again. But after this eye-opening consultation, we decide that we need to find a donor as soon as possible, and both begin trying each time we ovulate.

The more we learn about this process, the more we realize that all of the offers from well-intentioned men in distant yet intriguing corners of the world are impractical. We need someone within striking distance that we can call up whenever our trusty pee stick alerts us to the fact that one of us is ovulating. The timing on this is far more complex than I ever knew. Both Viviën and I have for the most part dated women and so hadn't had to consider fertility from the end of the spectrum that many straight women do — in terms of birth control.

There are two stages to a woman's cycle, we learn — the follicular phase (when the egg is formed) and the luteal phase (where it is fertilized or released) — and theoretically an egg will appear at the beginning of the luteal phase, on the fourteenth day of a woman's menstrual cycle. The egg remains fertile for between twelve and forty-eight hours before it begins to disintegrate. You can roughly predict when a woman will release an egg by subtracting the length of her luteal phase from the length of her cycle. The tricky bit, however, is that the length of this cycle can vary. Ovulation can be delayed by factors like stress, diet, physical activity, etc. What this means is that if your cycle is somewhat irregular, you'll need access to sperm on demand.

So it is with this new sense of urgency that we head out to meet up with The Lawyer of the meagre profile. I, for one, have resolved to like him no matter what.

"If he's a lawyer then we can be reasonably sure he's not an ex-con," I say.

"Do you think we're dangerously lowering our standards?" Viviën asks.

"Should we tell him we've been seeing other guys? But then he might not take us seriously. Maybe he'll start talking to other women. Then again, what if we do end up going with someone else? We're going to have to be honest about that. I want all of this to be on the up and up. We don't want to leave him hanging. We'll have to make a clean break so that he can get on with his life."

"Maybe we should just meet him first," says Viviën, ever the voice of reason.

That sounds great but I know if he asks me directly whether we have met with other potential donors, I will just blurt the truth. I'm among the world's worst liars, particularly at point blank range.

We walk into the appointed coffee chain at the appointed time and begin rubbernecking with that distinctive air of someone looking for someone who is looking for someone they haven't met in the flesh.

The Lawyer spots us and gives the tiniest of waves. When I return it and touch Viviën's elbow to direct her eyes to our "date," he gives a kind of shiver. I'm not sure what kind of women he is expecting, but his reaction seems to say that we aren't them. *I was hoping for someone else.* At this point I chicken out and dart toward the counter to get lattes, leaving Viviën to sit down with him and break the ice. From the look of things, she'll need an arctic class navy destroyer to do that.

As I make my way through the sluggish line, I can see Viviën shooting me desperate looks. This will be the last time I get away with the latte dodge. She leans forward, her brow furrowed. I can see the muscles in her neck getting tighter and tighter from across the room. Finally I get our order and head over to the table.

I extend my hand for a shake and begin to say, "no, no, don't get up…" then trail off when I realize he has no intention of standing. He shakes my hand from a sitting position, which in itself is odd, but he also has a most unfortunate handshake. His hand enveloping mine is cold, moist … almost amphibian. Imagine a handful of calamari before it hits the fryer. The hand is also alarmingly white and matches the rest of him in hue. He still hasn't released my hand, and I can feel little pins and needles along the back of my neck. I am just about to give my hand a little yank to dislodge it when he releases his grip and my hand slides out, damp. I have to stop myself from wiping it on my pants.

That must be a handicap in his line of work, I think. Don't lawyers have to shake hands all day? At least this is what my careful study of Hollywood movies has taught me. Light bounces off The Lawyer's pallid forehead and produces a glare that makes it difficult to look him in the eye. A thick, muddy, coffee-scented silence hangs over our table. I take a gulp of air and stammer, "Okay. Great. We're here. Thanks so much for taking the time to meet us. Did you have a good drive across town?"

A pause. All of his features contract into a knot — as if he is gathering steam for a courtroom rebuttal — before he painstaking answers, "It was … uneventful."

He listens as we describe our ideal scenario while swirling the dregs of coffee around in his Starbucks cup.

"As we mentioned we aren't looking for a full-time co-parent," I begin.

"But it would be great if our child, or children, could get to know their biological father," Viviën continues.

We try to remain upbeat and finish our pitch but he is unresponsive. He has remarkably little to say about himself and responds to our questions about him with one-word answers. When we ask him why he is thinking of being a donor, he replies that he is fifty years old and hasn't had a date for two years.

"At this point it is statistically improbably that I will meet someone, get married and have children the normal way," he says.

I rankle as he drops the word "normal" but hold back. His disclosures are taking us into frightening terrain. At that moment, we have no other local prospects, and despite the sinking feeling in my gut, I don't want to lose him. We need to somehow uncouple our endeavour from the entire weight of his disappointment … but life rarely works that way. Complexities complexify, is the general rule.

"Fifty is not late too fall in love and start a family," I offer.

"And be up all hours of the night? Babies are a lot of work, you know," he says, as if we might not have considered this aspect of child rearing.

"Well it's certainly not too late to meet someone and fall in love," I say.

"No. I have pretty much given up on that too," he mutters.

"Oh. But that's kind of …"

"Sad," he says. "It's sad."

Then I make the mistake of pressing him about his reasons for responding to our profile. Is he really fond of babies? Does he have nieces or nephews that warm his heart? No, he replies, he isn't particularly fond of babies but children are okay if they aren't too sticky or too loud. He responded to our ad, he explains, because it makes sense from the point of view of the economic concept of opportunity cost. This concept measures the cost of any activity in terms of the next best alternative that is not chosen, he explains. It is the cost/lost benefit of the foregone products after making a choice.

"I see, so in your scenario we would be like a kind of ..."

"Insurance policy," he replies with brutal honesty. "This way I can be sure I'm not missing out on anything."

"I see." Viviën looks out the window. That last is too much for her, I fear. Damp coffee scented silence reigns. Condensation running down the windows makes it look like the coffee shop is crying. I can hear crickets chirping outside even though we are in the heart of a concrete city block. *Cheep, cheep, cheep.* We sit there soaked by the harsh light and surrounded by questionably motivated prints of happy children picking coffee beans.

*Why did we come here?* I think to myself. *This place sucks the life out of everything.* I look over at Viviën, who is studying her shoelaces as if there is a complex algebra problem inscribed on them that desperately needs solving.

I want to stand up and dash. But we invited him here, and the laws of civility dictate that we must see this sad date through to its conclusion. I kick Viviën under the table, meaning *Your turn, you ask him something.*

"Ow," she says out loud, startled, then tries unsuccessfully to turn the outburst into a cough. "Do you have any hobbies?"

"I am a swimmer," he replies, and we try not to look doubtfully at his slumped over potato shape.

"I used to swim" he corrects. And then, after a moment: "I know *how* to swim, I mean I don't sink. This probably isn't going to work," he admits finally.

A few more uncomfortable moments ooze by as time dilates. The art deco clock seems to be melting Dali style, about to slide down the wall in a globular heap. Even though the clock must be too far away, I can hear the seconds shear themselves off from the minute — one by one — with a mechanical tearing sound.

Finally we thank him for his time and make our dejected way out to the parking lot to drive back to our place across town, once more without a viable prospect.

## 10. those Nobelists could never win a basketball game

Offers of sperm continue to pour in from far and wide, though very few from men within an easy car ride. A quantum physicist from Romania emails us adorable baby pictures of himself. In his profile he lists himself as healthy, fit and six foot two inches tall, with twenty/twenty vision. He adds that he has no family history of congenital disease and is willing to undergo fresh STD tests.

He is living in London but plans to move to the United States for a post-doctoral position in black hole physics and early universe cosmology. When I ask about his work he explains that he works on superconductor simulations and horizon visualization via embedding in flat space. In order to investigate the nature of dark matter he is proposing a new type of ultra-light particle that will form halos supported by the quantum uncertainty principle. Pretty tame, really, he says, compared to his older research. I have no idea what he is talking about, but those are *very* cute baby pictures. Via a chat program I ask him whether any of those strands of quantum physics he is working on offer solutions to our geographical conundrum, and he replies that in the not too distant future they just might … but a more practical solution would be for him to stop by and see us on his way to his post-doc. When we write back and let him know that we'd both like to try and conceive he is very enthusiastic. He does, however, have one small requirement for all of his sperm recipients.

The phrase "all of" would likely raise a red flag for anyone except a couple of lesbians desperate to get pregnant. It turns out that before he will give any woman sperm he needs to see copies of their advanced degrees, complete with transcripts. He requires straight A's. While he considers the spreading of his gene pool to be his gift to humanity, he isn't interested in populating the world with dullards, he says. After that he waxes poetic — for at least three paragraphs — about the fact that since we'll be conceiving at the same time we'll also both be simultaneously breastfeeding and so our house would be a veritable milk factory. We could even swap the babies back and forth. One of us could breastfeed both babies simultaneously, he enthuses.

Now we are all in favour of breastfeeding. We're not signing up to be missionaries for La Leche League any time soon, but we've read up on the advantages of mother's milk for infants in terms of bonding, nutrition, and a strengthened immune system. Speculation of this sort from a distant and exacting physicist, however, is another matter. His enthusiasm for the topic borders on the fetishistic. Not to mention the fact that I probably have a couple B's lurking about in my transcripts if he really cares to dig.

What cinches it for us is when, in email number eight, the physicist feels the need to admit that he's been lying to us in his profile. He, his sister and his mother all wear glasses, his father has high blood pressure, his grandfather is bald, and he is actually an even five feet in his shoes. But he does have a tall uncle. He is indeed a physicist, however, and he does still want to see all of our post-secondary transcripts. Thank you very much, but no thank you. Delete, delete, delete. *Sigh.*

That's when we notice the oddly inverse relationship between height and sperm donation. In some of our more desperate moments we had (despite Viviën's reservations) cruised the catalogue of anonymous sperm donors offered by Canadian clinics. An overwhelming number of the few men who want to donate sperm for altruistic reasons are short, yet there is an overwhelming demand for so called "tall sperm."

In Canada people cannot sell their genetic material. A man cannot be paid for sperm, just as a woman cannot be paid to donate an egg. Anyone who makes a donation does so for altruistic reasons. This means that there is a shortage, and so some clinics buy their sperm from the U.S., where donors are paid. For these reasons, there are no firm answers as to just how many children might result from one viable Canadian donor.

One sperm bank in Ontario has a severe shortage of donor sperm from donors over five foot seven. We are surprised to find that height trumps almost anything else: intelligence, looks, personality traits, even ethnicity. If this is true, life must be quite difficult for men of shorter stature. I simply hadn't realized the extent to which culture discriminates against the vertically challenged.

This inverse relationship is also evident in some of the reading I do on the history of sperm banks in the United States. Things are very different south of the border when it comes to sperm donation as the profit incentive changes everything. Not only can men (and women for that matter) be paid for their reproductive cells, they are also valued and devalued according to the often dubious logic that governs the sale of any product.

Hence tall sperm costs more than short sperm. An Ivy League egg or womb costs more than one that has been to a state college and far more than one that has never undertaken higher education at all, despite the fact that there is no evidence that any desired traits would be passed on to a baby conceived with this material.

This assignation of value is taken to its logical extreme in the Repository for Germinal Choice, a sperm bank founded by Robert Klark Graham that existed from 1980 to 1999 to gather donations from Nobel Prize laureates and other intellectually gifted men. The female recipients not only had to pay for the sperm, they also needed to have a verifiable IQ in the top two percent of the population. In the end, very few Nobel Prize winners ever donated, and Graham roamed the country hunting for what he dubbed the finest "specimens" of American manhood. He courted his marks with the energy and passion of a lover and personally collected and distributed his samples in the misguided hopes of strengthening and enriching the human herd. Oddly enough, he considered himself unfit to contribute. It wasn't his intelligence that was the issue, he noted. He dubbed himself unsuitable as a donor because he was too short.

A very large stone was thrust into the path of Graham's Nobel sperm bank when research revealed that it was not only the advanced maternal age of a woman that increased the likelihood of birth defects: the sperm of older men was also more likely to increase this risk. Most men were in their golden years before they received such distinguishing awards and by that time they were past their prime reproductive years.

Another problem, noted Graham in his memoir, was that nobody wanted to have miniature versions of the little bald professors, despite their much lauded IQs. It seems that tall was the new smart. Women wanted high quality sperm, first. They wanted health, height and physical ability, and they sometimes asked how smart the donor was. They more often asked what he looked like, and they *always* asked how tall he was. Even the founder of the Nobel sperm bank himself acknowledged the quandary in the fullness of time. "Those Nobelists," he was reputed to have said scornfully, "they could never win a basketball game."

## 11. why wasn't I born a lesbian

Choice was a buzz word in the suede bell-bottomed Joan Baez 1970s that formed the texture of my childhood. A woman's right to choose what happens or does not happen inside her own body was on the front-line of political and cultural debate. The very word for me still signals the discourses of freedom and rights of the era: the choice to live and love as you want, freedom from segregation, the freedom to choose whether or not you serve in the military, or even go into the family business.

Now that we have joined the ranks of the infertile, the word "choice" begins to slide around and change meaning. Of course we are different from the traditional couple with fertility issues, and yet our hearts will likely break along the same fault lines should we ultimately be unable to have a baby.

For this reason a kind of instant kinship wells up between me and the woman I sit next to at the fertility clinic. I am here on my own as Viviën and I booked ourselves for fertility tests at different times. We want to be sure that we are physically able to carry babies, since it requires such elaborate arrangements to try. The woman looks over at me with kind eyes. Sure she has Armani on her back and Prada tucked under her arm and I have Chuckie All-Stars on my feet and a backpack full of books under my arm, but in our differently clad chests burns the same bright little flame of hope.

We have the same hope but in a province like Alberta, where most fertility procedures are not covered, we do not have the same options. While a basic fertility test is paid for by Alberta Health, any treatments we decide to undergo are not. It costs roughly $1500 to purchase a single sample of frozen donor sperm. The price includes the process of having the sperm inserted into your uterus, storage and cleaning. The success rates vary from between five and twenty-five percent, and so it is rec-ommended that couples be prepared to shoulder the cost of ten tries in order to give themselves a reasonable chance of getting pregnant.

If we decided to go that route we would need to plan and put extra money aside. To me, it seems to be an excessive price tag for a resource that is renewable and widely available. Excessive, that is, until I heard the woman sitting next to me unfold her story. She of the Armani and Prada (she is so well put together that the apparel seems to form a protective modern armour) leans over and asks me with the conspiratorial air of a fellow inmate: "What are you in for?"

"A test to see if I am fertile. An egg count, I think they call it, " I reply.

"We tried for eight years before my husband agreed to be tested. You know how difficult it is for a guy to admit …" here she pauses and waits for me to chime in. I sense that she hasn't read me as lesbian, and although I have no problem coming out, I don't want to interrupt her flow so I just nod and let her continue.

"Well we found out that he was the problem. No, I shouldn't say it like that, he'd *kill* me — I mean he's not infertile, but his sperm have improperly formed tails so they don't make it. You know." Here she inserts a hand gesture that is a pretty graphic approximation of sperm wriggling their way up through the fallopian tubes.

"Ah, the tail. I see," I say. I didn't actually know that sperm could have problems with their tails. In fact, before we embarked on this journey I don't think I knew very much about sperm at all, but now I spend a good chunk of each day in fascinated contemplation. "So you're using a donor, then?" I ask.

"If only! Oh my god, if only it were that easy but he'd never raise another man's baby," she says, shaking her head, and I can't help but feel the friction between our two worlds. If I were to explain our situation would she still imagine that my wife and I would be raising "another man's baby?" Maybe it is just an unfortunate turn of phrase but language is telling and important. I can feel my body unconsciously begin to angle itself away from her and my muscles slightly recoil of their own accord. I suddenly remember that the newspaper in my lap needs urgent reading, but Mrs. Armaniprada has more to say.

"Now that we've identified the problem there's a different procedure they can do. They use a needle to extract his sperm directly. A needle in the testicle isn't any man's idea of fun, so he wasn't exactly eager."

"No, I guess not." I can't help wincing on his behalf.

"By the time I could convince him to go for it — it's expensive as well …" she says.

"How much? If you don't mind me asking."

"Not at all, it is 12,000 dollars or so."

"What?" I think I must have heard wrong.

"For the first try. And it didn't work. Because by the time I could

31

convince him to go for this procedure, I was thirty-nine and — how old are you if you don't mind me asking?"

"No, I don't mind. I'm thirty-seven." Age, money, we're getting into all of the meaty stuff now.

"Ah," she says, nodding. Suddenly I feel her eyes looking directly inside mine for the first time since we started speaking. As if she is taking some kind of an emotional temperature check. "Then you know what I'm talking about. By then my eggs had deteriorated to the point where they advised us that trying the procedure again with my eggs just wasn't worth it. There was a chance, but it wasn't a good one. So we had to find a donor egg. Then they take out one of my husband's sperm, slice the tail off and introduce it directly to the egg, which they then implant into me when I go into heat. Sorry to be crude."

"No, it's fine. So you're here to see if it worked?"

"Oh no, I'm here for another try. This is number four, and altogether it is 20,000 each time. Not that we're counting. I mean you can't put a price on motherhood, can you?" she says.

Here I want to interject that no you can't … but it seems that somebody has, but by now she is getting on to the heart of her problem.

"It's not the money, but the fertility drugs, well they are really hard on your body — you'll see, they just rip the guts right out of you — and visits to clinic every week, getting your hopes up each time. It can wear you down, you know?"

That I do know. I can see sadness pooled in her eyes. "Well I am crossing my fingers for you," I say.

"Thanks, I will for you too. So is your husband …" here she trails off, looks around, takes me in again and scans the waiting room.

"No, I'm no husband. I mean I *have* no husband."

"Doing this all on your own, you brave girl."

"Sorry, no. I am married. To a woman." It is almost as if I see a sixty-watt light bulb fire up directly over her perfectly coifed head.

"Oh for god's sake, of course. Is your wife trying as well?" I nod in the affirmative, and she continues. "You are so lucky, you have double the odds! Why wasn't *I* born a lesbian?" She peers upward, directing the question to the crown moulding above us or to a higher power — it is difficult to be sure. *Now there's a question you don't hear every day.* Her name is called and she gives me a little pat on the knee as she gets up to leave.

Here I was feeling that we have a rocky road ahead. Here I was feeling just the tiniest bit sorry for us. Now this conversation has helped put things into perspective.

Twofold note to self:

1. Always talk to people in waiting rooms.
2. Don't do self-pity. Someone else has always got it worse.

## 12. elevation is important

Just when we begin to give up hope of ever finding a donor in Alberta, we are contacted by The Man Who Built Banff. Banff is a rustic ski village in the heart of the Rocky Mountains that houses hot springs and lodgings for skiers and winter adventurers. You might recognize nearby Lake Louise, whose distinctive turquoise waters adorn postcards and travel brochures. The unique colour of the lake is produced by rock flour. The steady grinding and shifting of the Victoria glacier creates rock particles so fine that they defy the laws of nature and remain suspended in the glacial waters, reflecting light and producing that ethereal and luminous blue-green.

The village of Banff has a distinctive building style. Raw logs are skinned, sanded, and polished to a preternatural gleam. Moose, deer and bear tracks are pressed into concrete walkways, and antlers adorn the façade of every building. The downtown is friendlier to walkers and skiers than cars, which creep along at a snail's pace as pedestrian tourists, chunks of fudge or postcards in hand, claim the few blocks of the main street.

We arrive at the coffee shop five minutes early. No franchise this time. Partly to ward off bad karma we chose a locally owned business that serves steaming mugs of fair trade coffee in giant pottery mugs. At first we don't realize that the fellow who jumps out of a jeep and steps toward us is our guy. He is nowhere near the six feet that he had posted in his profile. I reach for my phone to ring his number and then realize that the man in nicely broken-in Carhartt pants and a down vest is indeed our potential donor.

We introduce ourselves and shake hands. I note his handshake, which is warm and strong, and his kind twinkly blue eyes with smile lines around them. Tight coppery curls hug his head, and there doesn't seem to be enough of his upper lip to come down over his teeth, giving him the effect of a constant smile. He surprises us with a dramatic move, sweeping his arm out and throwing open the door of the coffee shop while saying: "Ladies before gentlemen."

Despite the out-of-context gesture, the fellow himself seems warm and genuine. Viviën and I, unaccustomed to chivalry but anxious to make friends, try to go through the door at the same time. This produces a kind of logjam where we step on one another's feet and, I suspect, his feet as well. Though it is not the most graceful of entrances, this hardly matters because by the time we get inside we are all smiling. Already, things seemed to be going better than they had on our last three "dates" combined.

"So we aren't looking for a full on co-parenting situation," I say, launching into our pitch. "You wouldn't be responsible for the child or children at all."

"We just want to give them a chance to maybe meet or know the other person who helped create them," Viviën adds.

Without ever discussing it, and perhaps through repetition alone, we have honed our routine. We hand our story off to one another with the speed and ease of sprinters passing the smooth steel baton in a relay race. With each meeting we need fewer words to get our points across. Instinctively we have figured out which details need emphasizing and which to leave aside. I sit in a strange spot in the conversation, simultaneously inside of it, due to being so invested in the outcome, and also outside of it, as I can't help but admire my wife as she speaks to our potential donor. The stakes are, of course, very high as we have started to wonder if we will ever find the donor we are looking for in Alberta. Viviën is far from her home country (Holland), far from her chosen country (France) and operating in her third language — yet she projects ease and grace with every word.

Even though we are getting better all the time at delivering our pitch, we would really love to stop perfecting our opening act and get on to the main production. We both hope this fellow is the one.

The Man Who Built Banff responds warmly. He has a really good sense about people, he says, and he can tell that we'll be wonderful parents. That is certainly great to hear, but even more importantly seems to bode well for him depositing his semen in a sterile container on our behalf in the not-too-distant future.

We ask him about his family, and he pulls out a gorgeous photo — him and his wife, two teenage sons and a daughter on a powdery summit. Their goggles atop their heads and the sun on their faces, aglow with health and magnanimity, they are the quintessence of the happy family. His children, he tells us, are the light of his life: "I would love to have more. Heck, I would have ten more if I could. But I'm not the one who brings them into this world, that's the wife, so she's the boss." He throws up his hands up in a gesture of affable helplessness.

We ask how his wife feels about him being a donor, and he says that not only is she supportive of his decision, she thinks it is almost his responsibility to help other couples who can't have babies on their own (like us!) to start a family.

What a wonderful woman. What sensible and forward-thinking people. What open-minded humanitarians. My Maritime roots showing, I think: *who knew people like this existed in Alberta?* I give myself an internal dressing down for being so quick to judge the inhabitants of this beautiful province. Here are people who care deeply about the fabric of society: Compassion is alive and well in Wild Rose Country.

The Man Who Built Banff tells us about each of his children in turn: the bookworm, the star athlete and the future geologist. He enumerates their accomplishments and recounts heart-warming stories from their early childhoods. The joy they bring into his life is writ large across his face and animates every gesture. What does it matter if he measures far under his advertised height? This guy is the real deal.

In addition to loving anecdotes about his children, The Man Who Built Banff tells us how he and his Scottish ancestors hauled themselves up by their bootstraps. His own father, who lives in the muskeg of Northern Ontario, still walks his trap lines at the age of ninety-two. Longevity, determination and resourcefulness. No one really knows to what degree such traits are inherited, but we are seduced by the idea nonetheless. I am breathless with my own desire to pop the question. *Will you be our sperm donor?* I want to ask him, but know I have to let the dust settle on our first meeting first.

Finally, The Man Who Built Banff lays down his ace in the hole. He has what none of the other men we met or talked to so far has: experience. He has already been a donor. Now, neither Viviën nor I are shrinking violets, but no matter how you slice it, asking a near stranger to ejaculate into a cup for you provokes a certain amount of awkwardness. So, we are relieved beyond belief when he tells us that he's already made a donation to a female police officer in Calgary. That's not exactly what he calls her, however. What he dubs her is a ladycop. I wonder for a moment how she might feel about that moniker, but with even more force, I wonder if the procedure had been a success, and if so, whether she was gestating a wee babycop as we spoke. We are both eager to hear how the mechanics of the donation were arranged, and Viviën urges him to tell us about it.

"She thought it would be easier if I came to her so I brought along a fresh set of STD tests to put her mind at ease when I drove into the city. We had a little chat, a little coffee. Then I went into her spare bedroom and collected my sperm in a sterile container. I left pretty quick after that, because the sooner you get the stuff in there, the higher your chances of conception," he says and then adds: "Oh, if for any reason you can't insert it right away, carry the container next to your skin. Sperm need to stay at body temperature or they start to die right away."

We are impressed not only with his calm, easy manner but also with the depth of his knowledge. He seems to not only have been a donor but also to have read up on the process. Viviën asks him if the donation was successful, and we both lean forward for the answer. We want to know A) how potent our prospect's sperm is and B) whether our future children will have a little crime-fighting half brother or sister running around Calgary.

"The donation did not take," he says, shaking his head sadly, "most likely because she lost most of it."

"What do you mean lost it?" I ask.

"Right after you put the sperm in, you got to get your legs high up in the air. The ladycop, she just stood up right after and it all came right back out. Elevation is the key."

I make a mental note to stand on my head for at least an hour after inserting the semen … that is, if this kind man does, indeed, see his way fit to give us some of his sperm. Despite having never met her, I rankle at the carelessness of this sperm-losing ladycop. Unnervingly, she keeps appearing in my mind's eye wearing her tall black hat and half of her red ceremonial Mountie uniform.

I heave this hovering mental image aside and focus. The Man Who Built Banff is, he says, happy to get a fresh set of STD tests for us too. He is volunteering. Without us even asking, here he is offering to make our dream of having a baby a reality. With a family of his own, we can be pretty sure he won't change his mind later and want to play a larger role in our lives. He is clearly untroubled by the prospect of a two-mom family. It seems we have found the perfect donor. We imagine him telling our children the story of how he met us and decided to help us make them. We imagine him introducing our children to his own family. Perhaps a picnic or a barbeque in the distant future. There will be no mystery about their origin — only this wonderful man who had done us the most important of favours.

Deferring to his experience and wanting to make the donation process easy for him, we ask him what kind of arrangements he prefers. He confesses to having found it a bit difficult last time to relax and give a donation in someone else's home and wonders if we can come and stay overnight at his inn when the time is right.

Leaping at the chance to make things easier for him, we offer to call on the day we detect our ovulation cycle and then travel out to Banff. That way, he would be in his own environment and not even lose a day's work. He gives us a business card for one of the inns he owns. The picture on the card shows the building tricked out in the distinctive Banff neo-rustic style. Chinked log construction meant to evoke settler days. Settlers in the Canadian North would have been too busy fighting off scurvy and making shady land deals to ever de-bark, sand and stain each log so perfectly. That hardly matters, however, because we aren't going to stay long and we have only one purpose in mind. We part ways warmly and plan to try to get pregnant in January, when Viviën returns from phase two of our construction project in Nova Scotia. The Man Who Built Banff flashes us a winsome smile and we all get up to go.

It has been a long and intense conversation. Perhaps because of the intimate ground we've covered, it seems suddenly as if I've known The Man Who Built Banff for longer than one afternoon. This time when he holds the door open for me, I sail through effortlessly with the lace-chignoned ghost of Blanche Dubois fluttering away over my left shoulder. *That's it,* she breathes in my ear. *Ladies first. You must be adaptable to circumstances after all.*

## 13. Indomitable Lions

Another man has responded to our profile on free-sperm-donors.com. He is originally from Cameroon, but living in Calgary. We exchange a couple of cordial emails with some particulars covering the expectations each of us has. After I tell him that Cameroon's Indomitable Lions are my favourite soccer team, he agrees to a phone call. Soccer, or football as it is known in most of the world, gives us some enjoyable common ground to cover during the inevitable small talk portion of the conversation.

We agree that the return to the four-three-three formation was questionable at best and commiserate over the monumental loss to England in overtime in the quarter finals. So close, so close! Even though Viviën and I are reasonably sure that we already have our donor in The Man Who Built Banff, I figure it can't hurt to meet for coffee.

Also, while we are intensely grateful that The Man Who Built Banff is willing to give us sperm, he is also clear that he doesn't want to play any kind of role in their upbringing. He said he would not mind if they want to come and introduce themselves later on in life but he doesn't want to be a part of their lives in an ongoing way. We had become so caught up in the excitement of finally finding a willing donor and finally taking action on Operation Pregnant 2.0 that we kind of forgot about our ideal vision. Initially we pictured a man who would not have to parent on a day-to-day basis or make decisions about the child's life, etc. Rather we imagined someone who did not have children of their own and to whom playing a smaller role in the life of a child would be a boon. We envisioned a donor who would exchange photos with the children, come over and have dinner with us sometimes, and when the kids are older take them for the occasional outing. It isn't so much that we need help with parenting, just that we thought it was important for the children to be able to satisfy their curiosity about the other biological half of themselves.

This was our ideal, at any rate, and so I run it by Viviën to see if she thinks it is a good idea for me to meet with the fellow from Cameroon. She is still out east, working on our little ocean house, and plans to return at the end of January, when the renovations are finished. We talk about it and she says that she doesn't really want a donor who is a man of colour for herself, but doesn't mind if he would turn out to be a donor for me. For my part, since we are a mixed race couple, it might even be preferable. But then again, study all I want to about the concept of race, teach as I do the events of the civil rights movement … I will never understand colour the way she does, and so I absolutely respect her feelings on this count. This makes things complicated, however, because we also thought that it would be great if we could have the same doner for both of the children so that they could share a biological bond. These aspirations cut right to the quick of who we are and what we believe. We began with a utopian notion of how we could make a family but the deeper we wade into the experience the more we are realizing that we are going to have to be flexible. If we really and truly want to have a family then we might have to be very flexible; in fact we might have to let go of many or all of the ideas we had at the outset.

We agree that I should at least meet him for coffee before I leave to join her in Nova Scotia. If he and I get along, we can all three meet when she returns, and we can consider him as a donor for me.

He and I find each other without too much trouble, and after the obligatory commiseration about the weather — he tells me it was so cold when he got off the plane in this country he was sure the birds must freeze and fall from the air — he tells me about himself. He has a girlfriend with three small children, but they are not his. He runs an import/export business that brings goods into Canada from Africa for big supermarket chains. He speaks more French than English, so I explain our situation fumbling for words in my deeply flawed but serviceable French. He asks me what I do, and when I tell him that one of the subjects I teach is writing, he surprises me by dismissing the whole notion. He actually holds up one hand like a stop sign and says:

"No, this I do not believe. You cannot teach anyone to be an artist. A good friend of mine is an artist and he does it because he cannot help it. If you are truly an artist you don't really live in this world. You can sleep in a cave, you live in the street, eat sawdust if you have to, and you still care only for your art. It is a hard life. No one would choose this, and it cannot be taught."

He states this with such certainty that he shakes me up a little bit. Maybe he's right and I really am wasting my time in the classroom day after day. You can't give someone life experience in a classroom. You can't teach empathy, you can't light a fire in someone else's belly for them. However, if all of these things are present but dormant, you can certainly awaken them. This I do believe and I think I have done it at times. You can provide an informed community for the developing artist, and you can also give them a whole lexicon and a tool kit for editing and refining their work. Also he's using an overworked myth, in fact a cliché of the artist as a tortured soul living in a garret. I tell him so. He leans back in his chair and scratches his mini-goatee. I don't think he is used to someone forthrightly disagreeing with him, yet he takes it well, so I go on.

"The idea of an artist as a victim or a martyr is compelling because you do have to make sacrifices. But what about the joy to be found in making something out of nothing. First you have nothing, or rather, raw material. A hunk of stone, a lump of clay, a blank sheet of paper. Then, gradually, something begins to appear, to become refined. A voice rings out where before there was a silence. A spark! Recognition. We all have this joy, at first, as children. And then sadly and slowly we lose it."

Mr. Import/Export is listening but still shaking his head.

"Okay, let me put it another way. Let's just say that artists haven't cornered the market on suffering. Tell me, how many happy-go-lucky insurance adjustors do you know? How many sublimely content grocery store clerks? Blissed-out airport bathroom attendants?"

Now he cracks a smile and that's good enough for me.

I ask him if he would like to meet Vivien when she gets back and then think about being a donor for us. I am about to suggest a date when we can all get together and discuss the possibility, but he surprises me by quickly coming to a decision. If we want his sperm, he will provide it. I am somewhat taken aback but still excited. "Don't you want to take some time to consider?" I ask him. He says that these types of decisions, even by those making of a child in the usual way, are not matters of logic and consideration. We do these things by feeling. He has a good feeling about me and so he will do it. I ask him and he has no problem with going to the doctor for a batch of comprehensive STD tests. This, in turn, gives me a good feeling. We part ways with a very heavy sense of the maybe hanging in the air. I go home and talk to Viviën on the phone about him. She says she's willing to have coffee with him when she gets back.

## 14. (still) under construction

When I arrive in Nova Scotia I am impressed with all the renovations that Viviën has managed to complete in the brief time she's had. With help from one of my handy younger cousins she has studded in all the walls, upstairs and down, put in a kitchen and a bathroom, and mounted all the drywall. It is beginning to look less like a construction site and more like a home. Taking short breaks to eat lobster and raise toasts with family and friends, we nonetheless work like demons every day of the Christmas holiday. The more we get done together, the faster she can rejoin me in Calgary. We spend New Year's Day mixing concrete and pressing hunks of naturally flat shale that we found near the shore to form a base for the woodstove. This is an idea we conceived together and the result is ruggedly beautiful as well as functional. It comes out fine and mild, and we sit in the truck to eat our lunch. We have forgotten utensils and so eat with bare fingers. Folks out for a drive see us there and wave. When we began renovating this place, the guys down on the wharf used to shake their heads and smile. Two women alone on a construction site is an unusual sight back here, let alone two women firing up cement mixers, nail guns and welders. By now, however, they have become accustomed to us. We've been absorbed into the fabric of the little town. The town's mayor drives to council meetings either in his VW Scooby Doo replica van, or his red and blue Spider Man jeep bedecked with webs. There is guy who fills the back harbour with miniature ships that float up and down with the tide, and a rich American who bought an island off the coast and set up his own ham radio station. The town isn't short of eccentrics, but there is always room for a couple more.

Happy and exhausted we toast with what we have on hand — flat ginger ale — to what we've accomplished and to starting our family. I have to return because my classes start up right after New Year's, but Viviën will stay behind until the renovations are complete. We can't book her ticket until she starts to close in on the big items left to do, and it is so hard to leave her down there buried in snow drifts in a place that is home for me but to her must feel like the end of the earth. Meanwhile I go back alone to freezing cold Calgary, a city that neither one of us ever feels like more than a visitor in.

## 15. busted flat in Banff

When I pick Viviën up at the airport back in Calgary, I can spot her familiar walk all the way down the long corridor of polished tile. She has the solid stride of an athlete, and no matter where she puts her feet down, be it in her own country or another, a path in the forest or the crowded asphalt of a city sidewalk, you can tell she feels the earth. I wave and catch her eye. I know love makes fools of us all, and better poets than me have died, white knuckles gripping the edges of their Underwoods (or fountain pens or clay tablets), trying to capture the essence of this feeling, so I won't. Suffice it to say that the first time she looked at me my future began remaking itself around her. I knew I could never let her go. After we hold each other for a minute we head over to "odd/oversized luggage" to wait for our dog Rockit to emerge from the belly of the plane. He'd be so miffed if he could read. When he comes down the belt, he hears my voice and yips his indignation at being in dog jail. When we let him out, he goes crazy and covers me with slobber. We take him outside and he runs back and forth between us a few times until he's satisfied that no one is going to take off, then finds a spot, flattens his ears back and takes a long, much needed pee.

In the truck on the way to our house I give Viviën's leg a squeeze and ask her if she thinks her surge is coming. "Why," she jokes, "are you going to take me home and get me pregnant?"

"Always happy to try," I reply, with a wink.

The next day we start taking her temperature, but the thermometer proves useless for our purposes. You can detect your ovulation surge with a measurable spike in temperature, but you would have to be going off like Vesuvius for that thing to measure any marked difference from standard body temp. Instead we have to use the very expensive pee sticks that tell you exactly when you are ovulating. I wish I had stocks in the pee-stick-ovulation-detection company because as far as I can see it is just a little bitty piece of litmus paper, and at its price, the charge must be about a thousand bucks for a letter size piece of it. However, at this point, we don't care how many sticks we have to pee on. We have been in the planning stage for a long time and we don't want to miss an ovulation and have to wait yet another month.

So we watch the sticks for signs. Like some postmodern augury of good things to come we line them up on the bathroom counter. When ovulation approaches, the line in the little window is light at first, then darker and darker, each etching becoming more certain than the last. Because we are so anxious not to miss the surge and because even the "one day sooner" super-duper pee sticks are at best an imperfect science, we sometimes second guess it. *Is that really darker than yesterday or is it my imagination?* About a week into February, Viviën gets an unequivocal stripe — inky, assertive and so dark it has a shadow. This is convenient because it happens to be a weekend. I won't have to cancel class (though for this I would), and The Man Who Built Banff is likely to have a bit more free time as well.

Viviën and I have an agreement that the one who is being inseminated doesn't have to do any of the arranging. She doesn't have to make phone calls, book hotel rooms or even have to decide what to do for dinner if she doesn't want to. This is because we read that if you are relaxed and stress free, you increase your chances of conceiving.

It is a crisp blue day and, as often happens in Calgary, the sun beats down with such force that it fools you. You look out the window and think what a gorgeous day for a walk. Then you step outside and any skin you were foolish enough to leave exposed freezes instantly.

I call The Man Who Built Banff and tell him that today is the day: we have detected a definite surge! We will throw some things in a bag, stop at our favourite breakfast joint, and then make our way out to stay in his inn. As planned, we'll stay overnight so he can drop by whenever it is convenient.

"Ah, can we do it in a day or so?" he asks. I reply that actually we can't because the timing is very important. I'm a bit puzzled, because he seemed to know that was the case when we talked to him last. It's hard to believe, but if you really want to maximize your chances of conceiving you have to figure out when you are ovulating almost to the hour. He says okay then, come on out, and give him a call when we get here, but he sounds a bit less effusive than he did when we met him in person. He must be working pretty hard, I think to myself, and decide not to trouble Viviën with this. Phases Five and Six of Banff won't just build themselves, but he'll find a few minutes to fit us in like he said.

We are excited, almost giddy, the whole drive out of the city to the foothills of the Rockies. I wind down the window, and the dog and I hang our heads out the windows to drink in the mountain air until Viviën declares that we are going to freeze her to death. We are on our way! After all the planning and all the discussions we'd had about starting a family we are finally going to have our first real try at it. On the drive out, I am sure to play music that Viviën likes. She has some concerns about how we'll handle it, when the moment arrives, and we talk through it all so that she is as comfortable as possible.

"Hey, don't forget he's done this before," I reassure her. "The ladycop, remember?" Before we know it Barbara barks out that we're ten minutes from our destination and itemizes all the turns we'll have to make to arrive at The Man Who Built Banff's inn. Barbara is the name a friend of mine gave our GPS. If you're going to have a machine with a nasal voice telling you which turn to take, how fast to go, and generally just bossing you around all the time, you might as well personalize it, she reasoned, and the name stuck.

We pull up in the front of the inn. This is it. In a matter of hours we could be starting a new little life that will completely alter both our own lives and become its own little person with its own little destiny. I get out and take a deep breath. The air is even fresher out here than it is close to the city. From Banff you can see the rim of the Rocky Mountain chain slicing the horizon into a jagged line. Each mountain shoulders its impressive white cap. Even though we've been living out here for a couple years, this view still takes me by surprise.

The Man Who Built Banff sees us arrive. I say hello and compliment his place, although actually I think it is trying a bit too hard to be rustic. He seems distracted but says that he'll call us later and waves us toward the desk to check in.

We get our bags and make our way inside to the front desk, where the woman with a crisp dyed blonde bob fixes us with a venomous glare. "Who might you be?" she demands in a very unfrontdesklike manner.

I tell her our names, spelling them for her so she can enter them in her computer, all the while twisting my head this way and that, trying to see where our donor went. Why would he hire such a grumpy lady to work the front desk, I wonder. Then I take another look at the woman and something about her seems familiar. The family photograph! This is his wife. There is such a dissonance between the smiling woman in the photo and the teeth-baring hyena before us that I didn't even recognize her.

"That will be $189 plus tax for one night, and you pay in advance," she snaps.

"That's odd. I can certainly give you a credit card impression ... but every hotel I've ever stayed in, you leave a credit card number for incidentals and pay on the way out."

"That's our policy. If you don't like it there are several other inns just down the road."

I must be making a very strange face because Viviën, who is out of the sight line of the desk, catches my eye and mouths "What's wrong?" She hasn't recognized the woman and waits with the bags a few paces away. Maybe that's a good thing.

I have a feeling that something is off the rails here, but I desperately want the day and the donation to go smoothly. My biggest priority is to try and be a buffer for Viviën. I need her to stay relaxed and calm so that little egg she is making doesn't get stressed out either.

"It's okay babe, no problem," I say to her, and the woman's icy blue eyes dart up from her hotel ledger and stab mine. The look I encounter there is one that the life I've created allows me to largely avoid. I teach in a relatively enlightened and progressive work environment: the Canadian university system. I have a large and mostly supportive family, and I live in a country where — wonder of all wonders — I can live a full and equal life and now even get married. This is not the case in very many countries, and I don't take it for granted, but it means that on a day-to-day basis my relationship is given the ordinary amount of respect, and so I am completely unused to the evil eye the woman shoots at me when she hears me say "babe" to Viviën. It is loathing. Loathing combined with aggression and distaste. In short, her look is a big old nasty cocktail of bad vibes. I am so shocked that suddenly all I care about is getting Viviën away from this woman. I don't want her anger anywhere near my wife or the little egg she is cooking up in there, so I throw her my credit card the way you toss a raw steak to a vicious dog.

While she is processing the card, I rubberneck again but still can't spot The Man Who Built Banff, who appears to have melted into the Rocky Mountain woodwork. But we definitely need to have a word. Far from being supportive of his decision to be a donor for us, his wife seems opposed to us even staying at their inn. As she hands the bill back to me, she actually manages to give me a paper cut! Glancing down at my index finger I see a bright dotted line of blood spring to the surface. If she sees it, she pretends not to. As I bring it to my mouth she just keeps staring at me as if she is willing me to drop dead right in front of her.

We grab our bags and head up the one flight of stairs to our room. There are a couple of sullen teenagers cleaning in the hallway who glower at us and don't return our greeting. Relieved to be inside, we drop our bags on the sofa and look around.

"What was that?" asks Viviën. I was hoping she didn't notice anything, but she is keenly sensitive in social situations.

"That … was the wife," I say.

"What, it couldn't be," Viviën replies.

"And those guys in the hall, I think those were his two oldest sons." *Were they also a bit chilly? Or maybe I'm just paranoid now.*

"Where's The Man Who Built Banff?" she asks.

"I don't know, but this is too freaky. I'm going to call his cell." He picks up right away, but before I can ask any questions, he says he is very busy but if we would just amuse ourselves for the day, he'll give us a call later on to let us know exactly what time he'll be able to drop by and give us a donation. He suggests we go for a hike on the lovely frozen river. Seeing little choice at this point, we do. It is frozen, alright. Viviën really minds the cold, even more than I do, and so this is definitely not her idea of fun. Come to think of it, it's not mine either. We try to keep our spirits up and walk along, beating our mittened hands on our legs to keep them from going numb.

People swarm the streets of Banff shopping for ridiculously expensive pieces of slippery engineered plastic to strap to their feet and drink things that shouldn't even exist, like no-fat, lactose-free caramel macchiatos. Rockit is the only one enjoying himself. We throw a stick for him on the snow-covered bank while we are waiting. He plunges out of sight in the drifts and then re-emerges in another spot with frozen foam over his muzzle like some kind of rabid arctic dingo. After a while we are completely frozen and so even though we aren't hungry we go into a restaurant for an early supper. Despite the creative names on the menu, everything we order turns out to be both stale and expensive. Neither of us has the chutzpah to send it back, focused as we are on the task at hand, and so we sit there and pick at it, trying not to look at our watches. This isn't how we imagined the day, and there is something terribly un-restful about not knowing what time he's going to come over.

I desperately want to help Viviën relax because I've just read an article all about how your mood and your mental state can impact your body, especially at such crucial junctures of the ovulation process. If she gets all tense, the little egg might just call it quits. It might decide not to descend, or descend but then not be in the mood to be fertilized. Of course, eggs don't have moods ... my mind is just running in circles trying to keep busy because the longer we sit here, the greater the chances are that all of this fuss to come out here, all of this arranging could be for nothing. Six o'clock strikes and then seven, with still no call. We decide to go back to our room and wait.

This time, as we enter, I study the place more thoroughly. The wood isn't properly sanded, the tiles are cheap, and the workmanship is poor. You can only stomach so many rough hewn beams and oversized bear paw prints in the cement before you just wish people would move on and do something else.

We turn on a basketball game. The Raptors are winning but getting set to blow it in the fourth quarter as usual. It is getting late and it is very quiet. It seems as if we are the only guests, and the place begins to feel more and more like some twisted new version of the Bates Motel.

It's nearly eight when The Man Who Built Banff calls and says he is on his way over. I am relieved to hear from him, finally, but I register a note of tension in his voice. Five minutes later he knocks briefly, then steps inside looking positively funereal. He is a changed man. The ruddy apples have gone from his cheeks and all the power out of his chest. It is just as if someone found his air valve and let all the life out of him.

In another five minutes, I am supposed to be making love to my wife, inserting some promising genetic material and helping her to elevate her legs so that we can begin the next exciting stage of our life. Instead, I find myself consoling a straight man because he has brought upon himself the quintessential middle-class, middle-age disaster: he cheated on his wife with a younger woman and got caught. Yesterday. *Really? Seriously?* I just want to grab him by the ears and give his head a shake.

Now everything, even our innocently arranged and above-board donation, has become, in the eyes of his wife, part of his sordid behaviour. We listen and nod as the puzzle pieces of this odd day click into place.

His story goes from bad to worse, becoming increasing convoluted. It seems that in addition to being in the particular shit with his wife, his inn is in receivership as well. He loaned some money to someone a while back, on the honour system, and the fellow won't pay him back. Every week more notices arrive from the bank and creditors. He has been trying to hide it from everyone, not to worry his family about it, but now that he's been caught cheating, his whole house of cards has fallen down. His wife told him that she's leaving him, but if he makes a clean breast of everything and gets fitted with a GPS enabled microchip — maybe — just maybe, they could work it out. So that's what he'd been doing all day.

"So you mean you didn't tell her before that you were going to be a donor for us? Via *artificial* insemination?"

"I did tell her I'd have no problem doing that for someone, if the need arose."

"But she didn't know why we were here today?"

"No. She knew you were friends of mine."

"That's why she was so angry. Wait, friends? Don't you think you should clear this up with her?" He's really testing the elasticity of the word.

"It's no point telling her, she won't believe anything I say now…"

So much for making a clean breast of it. He crashes down in a heap on a chair. He wishes he could help us, but doesn't think that after the day he's had he'll be able to ejaculate, he says. Viviën and I look at each other. We are both very good in a crisis, but this type of situation is completely beyond our ken. We have no idea what to do or say, but it turns out we don't have to say anything. He needs, more than anything, to just sit for a moment and talk it out.

He can now see a pattern in the disasters in his life, he says. He tries to help people and it always gets him in trouble. He leans back and looks up into a chandelier of fifty watt bulbs as if an answer were written in the light filaments. *Not only are we not getting any sperm*, I think, *now we are ersatz marriage counsellors.* He goes on at length about how his life is in tatters around him. We are in a state of shock, so we automatically give some sympathetic response. I look at Viviën's face and see a huge amount of disappointment written there, yet here she is, still being kind and patient. Suddenly I feel like we need to get out of here at top speed. I begin to wonder if he might have been planning to ask for sex in return for a "donation." What a creep. I tell him we're leaving immediately, and he tries to convince us that it is late and we should stay the night. This is not going to happen. We firmly wish him the best and usher him to the door.

I get behind the wheel and we drive back from the Rockies toward the winking edges of Calgary, that ever-expanding pancake of light. The headlights pierce cones into the darkness. Viviën tips her head back as if for a little sleep and Janice Joplin comes on the radio. *Busted flat in Baton Rouge* — she grates out with her sandpaper voice — *waiting for a train, I was feeling near as faded as my jeans.* Our dog sighs audibly in the back seat as if he knows just how Janis feels. I reach over and put my hand on Viviën's thigh. Our cell phone bleats, and I grab it. Impossibly, it is The Man Who Built Banff.

"I'm sorry, but won't be able to reverse those charges on your credit card. Just give me your address and I'll send you some cash."

"What, why?"

He says that he doesn't want our refund to show up in the records because his niece does the books. We don't understand any of this, or why it would be a problem. Now it seems that, against our will, we have been woven into a fabric of secrecy that might ruin a marriage and tear a family apart. We wonder why he let us drive all the way out there and wait all day when he must have known that his life was falling apart. We don't know why he lied to us and his wife in the first place, and come to think of it, we don't even know what his real intentions were. All we know is that we feel dirty and used and hopeless as we drive back into town. All we know is that our hope of starting a family together, on this cycle, on this icy starlit night, have been firmly dashed. There aren't any strangers out there, it seems tonight, upon whose kindness you can rely.

Now Viviën leans her head against the window. She isn't sleeping but rather in the thick of a impenetrable quiet that I recognize as her way to salve a hurt. I would like to rage out loud and I can feel the burn of indignation in my throat, but instead I put my hand back on her leg and let it warm her through the denim. After another few kilometres she puts her broad, strong hand over mine and squeezes. "*Eikel*," she says. This is Dutch for asshole. "I don't want to think about it anymore right now. I don't want to think about it at all." She's right. We'll probably never get to the bottom of what just happened to us and it doesn't matter. Sometimes there is really nothing you can say to make it better. I take a breath and let it out, just let it out, along with my anger, to dissipate in the dark starry night.

## 16. house call

Mr. Import/Export from Cameroon is our next best option. We set up a coffee date and decide to go with Tim Hortons this time, hoping to dodge the Starbucks curse. Viviën finds Mr. Import/Export nice enough, although he seems more reserved and guarded than when I first met him. I am not sure why this is, but he speaks far less, and we run out of things to talk about fairly quickly. Although he is less talkative, he is still enthusiastic about being our donor and is even more interested when Viviën says that she'll also try to become pregnant using his sperm.

Since he is always travelling from one end of the city to the other for his business, he says it is easier for him to come to us than for us to find him. All we have to do is call him on his cell phone when we detect that one of us is ovulating, and he'll come right to the door and give us a fresh donation. This plan seems to be a big improvement on our last experience.

On the way home in the car we talk about it, and again Viviën says that he is not her ideal donor. Still here he is, ready, willing and able. Unless we reconsider our decision not to use an anonymous donor, he is our only prospect. I know, though she doesn't say it, that she is feeling the pressure. We had set ourselves a deadline of forty years old. Round numbers might not really mean much, but we do want to have enough youth and energy to give our children a good start in life. Time is running out for us, and so we talk ourselves into using a donor who might not be perfect for us but who is available. The most important thing, we must remember, is that a donor not pose any known medical risk to us or the children. We tell ourselves that if we were using a sperm bank, we would have no idea about any of these traits that we find so important now. How the heck would we know, if we went to the clinic and were inseminated with vial number 79948473, whether or not he would be good company at a dinner party? Also, I know that once the children appear we will love them very much, and we'll never be able to picture them any other way than how they are.

I burn through another box of pee sticks and finally get the dark solid line that indicates a surge in estrogen: I am ovulating. Vivien does the calling this time, and before long here is Mr. Import/Export, right on cue, ringing our doorbell. Our dog goes ballistic the way he does with every new visitor. He's not aggressive, just enthusiastic, but Mr. Import/Export looks alarmed. Where he grew up, he says, dogs aren't allowed in the house. We don't want to make him uncomfortable, and so Rockit is shooed unceremoniously into the backyard. Usually he would go and play, but now he feels slighted and sits by the glass patio door giving our guest the stink-eye.

We have downloaded a standard donor contract from the internet and give it to him to take a look at. He reads it over like a paralegal and, to my surprise, starts making radical changes. Some of them are minor but others make me uncomfortable. Especially the one he is most insistent about: he wants to be named as the legal guardian in the event that both of us die. He says he'll go out to his car and give us a few minutes alone to talk about the changes. If we're in agreement, he'll come back and sign it, and then he'll give us a donation.

I read his changes and they start to bother me more and more. "What if he is just having trouble finding a surrogate and so he'll wait until we give birth to the babies and then hire a hit man to bump us off?"

"Bump us off?" Vivien is looking at me quizzically. It's true, I'm probably consuming far too many detective shows. Vivien says that it is a good sign that he wants to be involved and that he is taking things seriously but I am not so sure. But at the same time, after so many false starts, we just desperately want to get going. I'm pretty much ready to sign about anything at this point, *just give me the darn sperm.* We invite him back, and he makes a series of additions and deletions that we initial until we have a draft that he is happy with. By the time we finish it seems as if we are about to create a new clause for the constitution, not a little human being, but finally the I's are dotted and the T's crossed, and the moment is at hand.

Viviën takes charge and directs him toward the upstairs extra bathroom for some privacy. We have laid out a proper receptacle, a fresh towel, etc. After he disappears up the stairs, it is so quiet that I dash over to the stereo to cover the silence with some music, but for the life of me can't come up with a proper entry into life's soundtrack for this occasion. Instead, I flip on the CBC, where Jian Ghomeshi and a learned guest, whose voice I cannot identify, are discussing the widening gap between the rich and the poor in our biggest cities and the erosion of the social safety net. I dart back toward the stereo but can't think what else to put on so I do a mad lap around the living room out of sheer nervous energy.

"Shh, he'll hear you," says Viviën and grabs me by the wrists. Suddenly we are both overcome with a fit of giggles. *There is a really a man upstairs in our house, really making sperm for us. Right now. We are really going to do this.* My stripe on the ovulation test was vivid and unquestionable this morning. Without very much ado at all, we hear the toilet flushing and the taps running. That was speedy. Mr. Import/Export comes down the stairs and slips himself into his snazzy leather shoes that he has politely left on the welcome mat near the front door.

I thank him, with a big silly smile on my face, and for some reason tackle him with something that starts out being a handshake and turns into a hug. What is the appropriate gesture with which to thank a near stranger for giving you a vial of his sperm? Blanche Dubois would know, I am sure, but she seems to have momentarily deserted me and I am left with my own slightly more rustic social graces.

Probably grateful to be untangled, he hops quickly into his sedan and wishes us luck.

"Thanks! We'll let you know as soon as we get any results from the pregnancy test!" I holler, thus giving our suspicious retired neighbour the last fact he needs for the file he is making on us either for the neighbourhood association or CSIS, I can't quite be sure. We are living in a rented townhouse in the foothills of Calgary, and to say that this is a quiet neighbourhood would be to vastly understate the case. We had our friends' kids over for a game of charades and a barbeque and got a letter from the condo board asking us to "cease and desist our public disturbances." We own a Toyota that's only a few years old and that we keep in good repair but we also got a letter notifying us that our "Old Truck" with its "noisy exhaust system" was disturbing residents.

The week we moved in, our neighbour was raking leaves and I was washing the truck, so I struck up a conversation. A hale and hearty man in his sixties, he leaned on the fence, grateful for the excuse to rest. He said that he didn't give a damn about the leaves at all.

"But the wife, you know, wants the yard looking a certain way." Here he jerked a thumb back over his shoulder toward their kitchen. "Just grow back again next year. A damn waste of time, if you ask me."

"Man, I know how you feel. Do you think I want to wash this truck? As soon as I go down the road, it's dirty again, but it makes the wife happy. Women, eh? Can't live with 'em, can't lock 'em in the kitchen." I was trying to break the ice and let him know that not only did he have lesbian neighbours, he had lesbian neighbours with a sense of humour. *Tada!* Didn't go over in real life the way it had, a few seconds before, in my head. That was the last time he spoke to me and, I think, the day he started the file on us.

As soon as Mr. Import/Export's tail lights disappear in the mist of his exhaust, we race upstairs to our bed. And this feels about as odd as it ever has. The thing is, if you are doing a home insemination, your chances are increased many times over if you actually make love, instead of just inserting the sperm. This is because the contractions from the orgasm of the partner being inseminated draw the sperm much further up into the uterus, at which point it has an eighty percent better shot at coming into the gravitational pull of the egg.

I remember my shock when, as an undergraduate, I encountered Emily Martin's groundbreaking article "The Egg and the Sperm: How Science has Constructed a Romance based on Stereotypical Male-Female Roles." Martin points out that not even scientific literature is free from prejudice. Despite clear evidence to the contrary, scientists almost invariably portray sperm as the initiator of life, the active party, while the egg sits patiently waiting to be penetrated. In fact, Martin says, the egg is very large compared to the sperm, and far from simply sitting there, the egg has a kind of gravitational force that actually pulls a sperm into its orbit, where it becomes stuck to the external coating of the egg, which then engulfs it. This does not deter scientific manuals, however, from skewing the facts in order to cause the sperm, despite their diminutive size, to loom in importance over the egg. In a collection of scientific papers, an electron micrograph of an enormous egg and a tiny sperm is called "A Portrait of the Sperm." Martin quips that this is a little like showing a photo of a dog and calling it a portrait of the flea! I found this article electrifying, not because I was interested in eggs and sperm at that time —in fact, back then these matters barely concerned me — but, rather, because it seemed to slice right to the heart of sex prejudice itself. In spite of all the wondrous things that science has given us, like vaccines for deadly diseases and electricity, scientists still explain their findings using metaphor, and the metaphors they choose necessarily reflect their own biases and also colour the results. Poof. So much for the myth of objectivity.

Now, of course, book learning is all well and good, but it still doesn't quite prepare you for the real thing. I have never actually seen semen in real life, and so I am very curious about the consistency and amount. What we have to me seems to be a small amount, about what you get when you blow your nose, but Viviën, who has only slightly more experience in this department than me, says this is normal. That strikes me as funny, and so I say the word out loud just to hear how it sounds. *Oh, I see, normal.* I hold the baggie for her while she sucks as much of the sperm as possible up into the needle-less syringe that we bought in its own sterile package at the drug store.

After she has most of it, I warm the vial between my hands. I don't want the sperm to get cold at all. This makes getting undressed rather challenging. My pieces of clothing get caught on one arm or one leg as I try to worm out of them while clutching the vial. I am trying to step on my sock with the opposite toe of the other and become completely entangled. Viviën has managed already to slide between the sheets while I stand here like some drop-out of the Houdini Academy. "Here," she says, and gestures to me that I should give her the vial. I pass it to her as if it were nitroglycerin, which, considering the changes it could blast into our lives and our bodies, is not an unreasonable simile. We lie together in bed, and it has to be said that heavy contract negotiations are not any-one's first choice of foreplay. Also there is the vial that we pass between us, being careful not to spill the contents.

However, once we are stretched out together our chemistry slowly creeps back into the room. Despite the somewhat forced circumstances of having to drop trou and make love on demand, the little white vial stays warm in my left hand. We find with surprise that it isn't as alienating as we thought. Because this experience is intense to be begin with and also because I'm a bit in awe over the change we are about to bring into our lives, I start to cry. This turns into laughter when Viviën remembers the only useful thing that came out of our trip to Banff: the advice to elevate after you insert the sperm. I walk my legs up the wall and she helps me stack pillows underneath.

"Why cry, I'm so silly," I say to her, my hand behind her neck. "It's still you. It's still me, after all."

## 17. the weight of each breast

When you want something very much, you begin to looking for signs everywhere. As I walk through the hallways at work, I nod and smile at colleagues and students as usual, but meanwhile I am wondering if I have a very important chemical reaction taking place inside of me. I notice pregnant women, even those in the early stages, whereas before I don't think I would have been aware of them until they were in the lower-back-clutching protuberant stage. I watch the way they carry themselves, as if mindful that they are a vessel carrying delicate cargo. Pregnant women seem to emit a kind of static electricity into the air around them. When I find one, I hang around and chat a while. Maybe her fertile vibes will rub off on me.

Viviën has her cycle once more and we try again with another help-ful donation delivered to our door by Mr. Import/Export. At this point either one of us — or even both, imagine! — could now pregnant and we wouldn't even know it.

It is still too early for even the most high tech pee stick in the world to tell us anything, so we are ticking off the days on the calendar and reading about the signs of early pregnancy. One of the clearest is supposed to be an increase in breast size. Of the two of us, Viviën is much more gifted in this department, and so I am kind of looking forward to it for myself. I could have cleavage. I could wear a V-neck.

Viviën tells me she's not a hundred percent sure but she thinks that her breasts feel heavier. Yippee!! This could be it. Unfortunately, in addition to the size increase there is also tenderness and pain. Is it wrong to ask "Oh, sweetie, do your breasts hurt" and when she says yes, to do a victory whoop?

"Let me see," I say and come over to check them out. She looks at mine and wonders if maybe they don't look a tiny bit bigger. She weighs one in each hand. Hmmm, hmmm. I am also examining hers. Yes, definitely a bit larger. When we suddenly realize what we were doing, we laugh and laugh: cupping each another's breasts in the middle of the living room, we are about as objective as two scientists.

## 18. eighty percent pregnant

Here comes the boy. He is five and crackling with energy, so his hair seems to stand on end. So many things catch his eye that he can't decide which to run after first and this is a mercy for his mother, who (two younger ones in tow) could never catch him if he truly made up his mind to bolt. As they move toward us, his limbs vibrate and his feet barely hit the sidewalk. The boy makes a kind of elliptical orbit around his mother, peppering her mercilessly with his questions:

*How many feathers does a bird have on each wing?*

*Who invented balloons?*

*The sky is blue and the grass is green … so what keeps the colours from mixing together where they touch?*

His queries are so beautiful they do not need answering; they hang in the air and exist for their own sake. He has a fist full of leaves in one hand, a fist full of twigs in the other, his chin tilted up to drink in the sky. Here comes the boy looking very much like my own, the one I keep seeing out of the corner of my eye. Yes here comes the little boy I imagine we could have if we ever do manage to have one.

At the sight of him, my wife ducks inside a store and walks, with purpose, toward the baby basketball sneakers. Naturally the first thing our children will need to learn upon arrival on this earth is to properly square their tiny shoulders and bend their knees for a jump shot.

"We said we wouldn't buy anything until …" I am superstitious and try to remind her of our agreement but find myself talking to the empty pocket of air where she stood one moment ago. Instead of shoes she's picked up a tiny package of fuzzy gray socks with blue stripes. Printed on the bottom of the feet in rubber (for grip) are the words: *It's mine, It's mine, It's mine*. When she heads for the checkout this time I don't have the heart to stop her.

On the way home in the car I ask if she feels anything out of the ordinary.

"I feel about eighty percent pregnant," she says, and I want to pile on the brakes, pull over to the side of the road, and circle the car in a loopy dance of joy… and I would do this, if we weren't heading into the curve of a large traffic roundabout.

"Eighty percent!? That's amazing! That makes me two hundred and eighty percent happy," I say and continue driving in my calm and cautious way.

"And my breasts hurt so much I feel like I need to hold them in my hands as I walk along."

"Babe, that's awesome!"

"Easy for you to say."

"I'd be pleased to hold them for you, any time at all, just say the word."

"You keep your eyes on the road," she says, smiling.

Out the window I spot the luminous ring of a sun dog on the edge of the prairie and take that for a good omen. What if it's worked? What if the little swimmers have found their egg inside of her and are getting on with the business of making our baby right now? What if the spinning supernova of the egg has attracted a sperm into its orbit. Key chemical reactions could be happening inside of her at this very moment. For that matter, they could also be happening inside of me. What if those important little cells have sorted it all out, found a spot that suits them, and are snuggling in to begin the exhausting work of dividing and subdividing until they make a baby. Or babies. If we both have a baby, they could grow up together, even be in the same class. Like twins. Sort of.

We have a pee date for Friday. Not the kind of Friday night date we're used to and perhaps an early intimation of how our lives are set to change. We are going to pee on a stick together and see if either of us has managed to get pregnant. It goes without saying that no matter which one of us carries the baby it will be ours, just ours, and that is all.

## 19. out damn spot

Viviën gets her period. This is really disappointing, especially after her feelings of eighty percent pregnancy. We are about to have a nice dinner with glasses of fruit juice mixed with soda water, our beverage of choice these days. There is only one more day to wait until we can test to see if we are pregnant. In the midst of mincing ginger she drops the knife on the cutting board and dashes to the bathroom. When she emerges the storm cloud over her strong and beautiful face tells the whole story: she won't be needing the pee stick on Friday.

To say we're devastated is an understatement, even though everything we've read confirms that we should expect to spend from six months to a year getting pregnant. But it just isn't as simple for us as it is for fertile straight couples. Like many other women trying to get pregnant, we begin by peeing on sticks to try and catch the first moment of ovulation. But when we get a positive, we have to contact our donor and hope that he is not working, out of town, or otherwise occupied. If he is not available, then we have no choice but to wait another month and try to orchestrate the whole thing again. The more we learn about conception, the more we understand the importance of timing. Although technically most women ovulate for several days, it is really the first few hours that hold your highest chances of conception.

Each time we find a willing donor, we are very grateful but also a little bit afraid that we might lose him. And it's no wonder. It wasn't easy to find a stranger willing to provide us with copies of tests showing he is HIV negative and free from STDs. No, it wasn't at all easy to find a man who, without wanting anything in return, would come over to our house, ejaculate into a cup and leave us with his sperm. He has done this twice, cheerfully, but it is the nature of a favour that it is something of a special occasion. I am unsure how many more times we can depend upon him to help us.

So we wait and wait. Time becomes elastic. How could every single hour take so long to tick off each interminable second? Tomorrow. Tomorrow we can try a test. Any earlier and we might get a false negative. The internal focus on something so important is difficult to manage at work. When people speak to me, I take an extra second to respond. Their reactions tell me that I must read as distracted or sedated ... or both, but it's not at all that I'm disinterested in what they are saying. Rather, I feel as if their voice is floating down a tunnel and into a cavern where I am waiting for a very important biological message.

Usually it is a joy to step into the classroom. I love the swapping of ideas and the gregarious exchange of intellect. I love being kept on my toes, antennae quivering for the next interesting turn in the conversation. I don't usually feel an effort to get myself to that state but now I do. Each time I feel as if I am grabbing a rope and cantilevering my psyche up out of its winter den.

## 20. endgame

I peel open a home pregnancy test and read the directions several times beginning to end. No, it's not rocket science, but I am new at this and want to be sure I get an accurate reading. The directions recommend holding the stick "mid-stream" for three seconds or catching the urine in a container and then immersing the stick for ten seconds. The first option seems challenging to both my balance and the laws of physics and so I opt for the second. I dip and count ... *one Mississippi, two Mississippi* ... to ten, then place the stick on the counter and stare at the little window where the x will appear if it is positive. I stare and stare at it some more. *Come on*, I breathe, but nothing happens. Water won't boil while you watch it, either. I turn away. I'll do something mundane, like look for friends for odd socks. I search for a few moments, match up a pair, give up on a couple more … then, without warning, pounce around the corner. Aha! A faint but ever darkening x is slowly appearing in the little window. It gets darker and darker, emerging from whiteness the way faces used to on Polaroids. x marks the spot! Buried treasure! I let out a whoop and Viviën comes running.

There it is. A lovely little purple inky x. A positive test on our first try. This is unbelievable considering the statistics the fertility doc threw at us. She cautioned us so sternly not to get our hopes up and to be prepared to keep basting ourselves with sperm for half a year at least. I show Viviën the stick and we grab each other around the waist and jump up and down like two schoolgirls. She lifts me up and I can feel the air rushing all around us as if it were a crisp wind of portent from the future. "Here we go," she says.

Now we dash over to the baby section, pick up onesies and tiny little shoes. We show them to each other and say "awwwww." I fight the urge to accost strangers and blurt out: *We're gonna have a baby*! Right into their startled faces. I search my appetites hoping to uncover bizarre cravings. Sardines and ice cream? Could I eat that? Artichokes with peanut butter?

It is not far along in the pregnancy when I am walking down the hall at work and feel something peculiar in my belly. I dart into the bathroom and find a spot, just a very tiny spot, but a spot nonetheless of blood. This isn't supposed to happen. I still have twenty minutes before I have to lecture and so I dash into my office, close the door and start researching what this could mean. *Light vaginal bleeding is common in the first trimester of pregnancy and need not be a sign of problems.* I read, with relief. *Persistent bleeding in the form of a steady flow, however, can be the first sign of miscarriage. Studies show that anywhere from 20–30% of women experience some degree of bleeding in early pregnancy.* Ah. I settle into the statistic feeling a bit safer but then I read on: *Approximately half of pregnant women who bleed have miscarriages, and the majority occur during the first 12 weeks.*

Where am I now? My brain works furiously as I try to situate myself numerically. What is this, week ten or eleven? The display on my computer blinks me a warning that I have to be in class in five minutes. Luckily my lecture today is on a play I've taught many times because I feel that I am about to do what I have never done yet in my career: teach on autopilot. Perhaps I should cancel the class, but I won't know what to do with myself anyway. I am teaching *Endgame* by Samuel Beckett. The endgame in chess, as you'll know if you're a player, is the final stage of the game where few pieces remain. Barring an unexpected error, the side that is strongest at the beginning of the endgame wins the match, so there is little to do but play it out to a foregone conclusion. Like many of Beckett's characters, Hamm and Clov are locked together in a mutual existential crisis. I figure I might as well put on a maxi pad for insurance, then get in there and duke it out with them as they search for the courage to end it all while buffeting each other with jabs of mutilating ennui.

I somehow manage to gain my footing in the lecture although my mind is racing and I am very afraid of what might be happening inside my body. With each word it gets easier, and despite being mortally distracted, I am still delighted by each nuance or bits of new meaning the students unearth in the text. Wanting to illuminate a passage for close reading, I bend over to flip the switch on the overhead. I feel a stab of pain as we examine the passage where Hamm tries to figure out what to do with his ailing parents, who somehow hang on, refusing to die, though they have no further joy in life.

HAMM: Sit on him.
CLOV: I can't sit.
HAMM: True. And I can't stand.
CLOV: So it is.
HAMM: Every man has his specialty.

I clear my throat and blink. I try to push down the sting I feel behind my eyes as I explain that Beckett's characters are not mean spirited. Beckett was trying to reflect a post World War Two world in which all major systems of meaning were collapsing. His characters make us confront the fact that a fully satisfying rational explanation of the universe is beyond our reach. That the very body that carts us around and the brains we are thinking this thought with are but pieces of gristle meat and bone in the process of dissolution. This requires people to take responsibility for their own actions and shape their own destinies. This realization is at once a source of despair and of profound freedom.

A student in the second row gets the lightbulb look and shoots her hand up.

"So … in other words, if your life sucks, there is no point to blaming someone else. It's all on you?"

"Yes," I say, "you've got it." My stomach is now in a vicious knot, and I feel a familiar trickle, then a flow. Tears well up in my eyes and there is a pause. The students gape at me for a moment. They stop texting, making notes, doodling, daydreaming. OMG, *the prof is crying. Awkward.*

As the class ends I know I need to get to the nearest bathroom, but one of my students intercepts me. She wants to do her honours paper on *Endgame*. She had always thought of Beckett as interesting but dry and bereft of emotion. She tells me, however, that during my lecture she accessed layers of hidden feeling within the hard shell of pessimism that she hadn't been aware of before. She fleshes out her idea. Her hands fly through the air as she draws the scaffolding that she is on fire about and that clearly has potential, and I tell her so. By now I am too afraid to go to the bathroom. The student walks a few steps toward the door with me, then heads off happily scribbling a note with a tiny metal stylus on her i-thing.

I don't even go back to my office for my jacket and things. I have the car keys and that's all I need, so I just push through the glass doors bare knuckling my stack of books against the knifeblade of the Calgary winter. I step quickly to the car, trying to clench muscles inside and willing the fragile little creature in there to please stay put. The slush has frozen into ankle-twisting ruts. Each stoplight takes about an hour as I sit in my car looking straight ahead. The tires of all the huge trucks around me are about level with the roof of my car, and sandwiched between them, I chant in time to the throbbing rhythm of their engines: *stay, stay, please stay, stay, stay, please stay.*

Viviën meets me at the door and I must look like hell because she looks afraid. There is a river of snot on my face and a river of blood in my pants, and all I can do is curl up in a ball on the sofa. I want to shut out the whole world and I know it isn't fair. It is her baby too. Could have been.

When I finally get up and go to the bathroom a few hours later, I am shocked to find something that looks almost exactly like a baby bird that has been taken too quickly out of its egg. There is the very tiny blue eye socket. There are the dark little masses of organs. Is that a liver, a kidney, a lung? The tissue surrounding them is delicate and veined like the flesh of a peach. I hold it in the cup of my palm. I realize I am completely out of my depth. I don't know what to do with this. This flesh, or this feeling. It is so borderline, this little life that could have been. I know it is too early to really call this a baby. I know that people might say I am lucky: if you are going to miscarry, it is better to do it early. I know they might tell me that there must have been something wrong with the baby and this is nature's way of taking care. I know they'll say that it doesn't mean I can't still have a baby later. I know they'll tell me this happens to women all the time and that it's normal, but it doesn't help.

I feel as if I have let everyone down. This feeling bears no relationship to logic and so also can't be touched or dispelled by it. I have let Viviën down, I have let our families down, and I have let this little creature down. Somehow I came up short, I was not a good host. Or worse, my body has let me down and now I hate it. I've always thought of my body as a sturdy and stalwart container: a reliable vehicle. I follow the owner's guide, fuel and oil it when necessary, don't subject it to undue strain, and generally expect it to take me where I want to go. Now it is a traitor. If your own body can betray you from within, then nothing is safe. Now anything goes. If my own womb can eject the little being we treasure so much, how do I know other body parts won't turn on me? I could awake in the night being strangled by my own hand.

I read as if words are bread and we are in a famine. I'm trying to figure out if there could be something wrong with me that would cause this, something I could do differently next time. I read online articles from medical journals. I read statistical analyses from fertility clinic websites. I read with mounting horror the heartbreaking things that have happened to other women during their pregnancies. What an ocean of pain. I had no idea. I read the blogs of women struggling with infertility. I log on to their forums and read their words as they vent and pray and search for answers. I read, but I don't write. I can't. Not a word, not a poem, not one line of dialogue, not even an email to a friend. This is something that has never happened to me. For the first time since I picked up a crayon and scrawled "once upon a time" in a campfire notebook, I have nothing at all to say.

It is Viviën who tells me to keep going. It must be easy, she says, to write when things go well. It is just as important to keep going when they don't. And she is right. The words just scampered all by themselves onto the page when we were flush and excited about our new brilliant plan. It is something else to write when I consider that this could be the story of how we tried to have babies and failed.

Having given so much of my life to writing, I wonder if it will let me down now. Maybe this devotion to the writing life is responsible for eating up so much of my life that I am only now starting to want all those things others want. A family, connection, continuity. To pass something on, other than words on a page. To watch my own colours fade gradually as new ones appear in a natural succession.

We've waded deeply in. We've let ourselves imagine … and now we have to say goodbye to an almost daughter or son. If I'm not able to be a mother, I could become one of those wistful people with the hungry eyes: the ones who know in their heart that they had it in them, that they wanted it and didn't manage to. When we decided to have a family together, we just assumed that we had all the time in the world. We thought it would be no problem to find someone, a friend or an acquaintance, who would be a sperm donor for us, help us start a family and play a role in our children's lives later on. We had something like a logical two-year plan worked out. Viviën would try to conceive first because she's a couple of years older, then I would have a baby a year or so later. The reality is much more complex and there are so many aspects that you can't control. In fact, maybe this process is all about the loss of control. Maybe that is its essence.

How could this happen? I thought I was seizing the day by travelling the world, making art, living in rehearsal spaces and changing cities every year. While I was busy seizing, is it possible that life itself, the new shoot that could have sprung from me, is dead at the root? Perhaps now even the writing life that I've so cherished will be as ashes in my mouth where before it was the ripest fruit. Wouldn't that be a sucker punch? Maybe that's exactly what happens when your reach exceeds your grasp.

## 21. there's the rub

It is a bit difficult to break it to Mr. Import/Export that neither attempt has been successful. I do my best to explain that this is normal and to have it work on the first attempt would have been beyond lucky. Still, I can feel his disappointment through the phone. It is recommended that you let your body rest for a bit after a miscarriage, and even if I wanted to try again right away my cycle is taking a while to find its equilibrium. Vivïen, however, is ready. I tell him this quickly because I sense that we might be losing him. We don't want to think about starting again from scratch with looking for a donor, and so I am quick to assure him that we'll have another chance in a few days. Another package of ovulation test sticks has determined that Vivïen's window of fertility is approaching.

Just as he promised, Mr. Import/Export arrives within a few hours of our call. For some reason it seems even stranger to usher him out this time. Since we've already run through all the preliminaries, this time I kind of feel like I'm giving him the "Here's your hat, what's your hurry" treatment. I don't mean to, to be sure. I appreciate social graces and good manners as much as the next girl, and I very much appreciate his coming over to our place and making the donation easier for us, but I don't want the sperm to get cold. He seems busy as well and happy to hit the road with a minimum of chat.

I find myself wondering just how much of a routine this will become for us. I have read of couples trying every month for a year or longer. We will do this if we have to, but I feel uncertain that any donor would want to stay the course for that long, unless they are very invested in having a child. I am still in a place of doubt about Mr. Import/Export's feelings on this front. He has been very accommodating in terms of providing his sperm but is still resistant to talking about what part the child or children might play in his life. He also completely stonewalls me when I ask him about the children of his girlfriend. They are still very small, all under five years old. They are not mine, is about all he will say, and this unnerves me. Of course, he has a right to his privacy, and I didn't expect that we'd all necessarily be having a family picnic together after a single sperm donation... But then again, why not? I am getting the feeling that he hasn't told his girlfriend that he is helping us try for children. This makes me nervous as I don't want any secrets of this nature in my own life, and being entwined in one, even peripherally, seems wrong, especially when it comes to as joyful a thing as making a baby. We are not going to push him on this front, however. Obviously not, we might lose our donor.

And so secret or no secret, girlfriend kept in the dark or not, we are still eager to have his sperm. I definitely feel commonality with those women who are buying sperm, buying eggs, paying someone to be a surrogate for them ... and the list goes on. Sure, you could be high minded about it. You could condemn such behaviours and compromises, but until you are in the position of wanting to be a parent — really committed to it — and then discover that you might not be able to, you can't judge. That's where we are now. I remember thinking to myself at the beginning, I would never take fertility drugs, I would never pay someone to be a surrogate ... now I don't know where the line is. I don't know what I could say "I would never" about. I want to have a baby, two if possible. I want to have a family.

After Mr. Import/Export leaves, Viviën and I get ready to make love "on demand." This isn't easy in the middle of the day when you know you have tasks ahead of you. This afternoon I must go to a meeting to draft a new vision statement for our department. Viviën, meanwhile, has to complete paperwork for her residency permit. With a heady cocktail of academic verbosity and bureaucratic red tape waiting for us it is little wonder that we're having a bit of trouble getting going. Add to that the fact that we are also having some real friction in our relationship for the first time since we committed to one another. Some of it is likely the difficulty we went through in finding a donor and the disappointment of the miscarriage, but there are other things that are totally unrelated.

First of all we live in Calgary. The Canadian prairie is not where I ever envisioned myself. I find the climate unforgiving and the landscape lacking, well, an ocean. For Vivën, already uprooted from Holland and the South of France, moving to Canada must have felt like a hardship posting. In fact she has told me this is the case, though using different words. Also, although I am trying, I am not learning Dutch nearly fast enough. I have picked up enough to be a source of amusement to a bright kindergartener, so this means most discussions default to English. Not fair, I know. It must be so alienating to be where no one speaks her language and to have to communicate even with her partner in a foreign tongue. I can't fix it, can't change it. All I can keep offering is that I love her fully, unconditionally, helplessly. If it all gets too much for her, I've told her, we can leave here. I'll follow her to Holland, France, wherever she wants to go. I'll go with her and try being the stranger.

The Dutch grow up learning several languages. This is practical in Western Europe as you travel a couple hundred kilometres and you need to speak a different tongue to communicate. Not so here in Canada, unfortunately, where we have English, English, a bit of French and more English. Before meeting her I couldn't even say good morning or thank-you in Dutch. The sounds and the alphabet all seemed awkward. Even when I can remember the words, I mispronounce them so badly that they are unrecognizable, and I feel like a dullard. I would love to study it, to have time to focus on it. I know it is important, and I want us to be able to speak both languages to one another, but right now it feels like we're just struggling to compose a life together. I am teaching full time, which, as a writer I find less than ideal.

We were both in the middle of renovation projects when we met, and as we try to finish them, each summer finds me with a hammer in my hand, not a pen. I feel maxed out so I have to admit that I haven't made learning Dutch a priority. After creating a family, work commitments and writing, Dutch comes in a distant fourth. Maybe it's not good enough, but for now I can't seem to wedge in a moment to work on a play or a poem at all. I try to explain why, even in the midst of everything we are trying to do, I have to keep working on writing projects … and end up sounding like a shallow jerk who wants to live on a desert island with a bunch of books and a typewriter.

Aye, that's the rub for most writers. We all want enough distance from the demands of life to allow us time to write about it, and yet if we build ourselves a sufficiently deep moat, in the end, no one will get across it. We will be so safe from the demands of life that we'll chase away the most vibrant and vital parts. We'll shut down the brightest chambers of our own heart. This, I am sure, I don't want.

Still, this friction over my Dutch (or lack thereof) isn't enough to drive a complete wedge between us. We race up the stairs, scattering a trail of clothes behind, and catch one another's eye to smile at our haste and acknowledge the silliness. Once we lie down, in spite of the hurry and the awkwardness of making love with a vial of sperm in one hand, it is still beautiful. In fact a little light bulb goes off in my head and makes a connection that I think successful couples have been making through the ages: when we don't get it on, we pick on one another. Bingo! I know it seems obvious, but I swear I had never made this link as cohesively as I did making love with my beloved wife, while hobbled by Mr. Import/ Export's sperm in my left fist to keep it warm.

I have to admit that I haven't felt very sexy at all in the last little while. Having a miscarriage and the heavy bleeding that followed made me just want to put a "closed for repairs" sign down below. It feels as if that part of myself has let me down and so I don't trust it. None of that is Viviën's fault and as soon as I look in her eyes or feel her soft warm skin against mine everything feels right. Yes, I just look in her eyes and all the good feelings just flood back in. All I have to do is let them.

## 22. better than no sperm at all

After finally getting my inner workings back on track and going through more expensive pee sticks than you can shake a … pee stick at, on Sunday morning, I finally get a measurable surge. We call Mr. Import/Export and though we have noticed a bit of a cooling off over the last months with each unsuccessful attempt, we are still hopeful. This call makes it clear that the sperm donor honeymoon is definitely over. Peevishness oozes through the phone. He says he might not be able to do it today because he's busy and plus, he doesn't feel good. He's tired and cold. He says maybe he'll change his mind and call us later in the afternoon. I feel a sinking in my stomach. Tired? Cold? Sheesh. I wonder how I'm going avoid tying myself into a knot of stress.

Viviën and I agree that he sounds distant. The carelessness with which he treats our phone calls is a concern. Of course I understand that this is all voluntary and of course he can change his mind about being our donor at any time, but I just wish he would be honest with us. I wonder how many women still manage to conceive a baby while their blood is secretly boiling in anger against the person whose sperm has been inserted into them. Then again maybe none of that matters. Probably lots of wonderful kids are conceived that way. Anger is a natural phenomenon, and perhaps it is to be expected to show its face when the stakes are so high.

I try to reason through this. I try to remember that he didn't promise to be our very own sperm-o-matic machine. I don't want to mechanize him, or be insensitive, and I don't want to scare him away. I wonder what he is thinking. And I keep on wondering because he doesn't call for the rest of the day, or half of the next. The window is closing. I can feel the egg inside of me waiting … waiting … checking its tiny wrist watch. Tapping its little toe and looking up and down at the silent street. Watching the street lights switch on. And finally calling it a day and sadly packing up to go home.

At eight o'clock we can't wait any more and so we call him. He doesn't pick up. We leave him two messages. I mean you're sick, fine … but at least let us know that you'll try in the morning or next month or whatever. The next day still nothing. I call about 10:30 — by now my surge is barely measurable, just a faded line shows in the window of the pee stick, where before there was a dark purple band. It would likely be a waste of time to try now. This makes me panic, not over losing this particular month, but because now I feel like I can't trust him. When he finally contacts us he gives a couple of conflicting stories about why he didn't call us back. Great, he doesn't even care enough to sort out a comprehensible lie, I think. I wonder why he is doing this at all, but at this point we don't have anyone else to help us.

He says he'll be home in the afternoon and if we drive over to his house in the far northeast of Calgary, he'll try to make us a sample. We pile ourselves in the car, wanting to try anyway but what with my faded ovulation line and the jumbled stories he's given us, my enthusiasm for doing this is about what you could conjure up for a rousing afternoon of dental surgery. But we committed to this and don't want to give up.

We drive over to his house in the suburbs. I have no idea who was in charge of the planning on this subdivision, but it is a symphony in beige. Light brown and taupe with identical townhouses as far as the eye can see. Who, I wonder, against the backdrop of the bald prairie, sits down and thinks: *I know just what this landscape needs, more beige.* Rows and rows of identical houses with tan plastic siding! Combined with the uniformity of the street names, a body could wonder lost forever as though stuck in Dante's fourth ring of hell. You drive down Oakview

Street to the corner of Oakview Green, closely followed by Oakview Glen, Curve, Street, Avenue, Square and Boulevard. All around, the brown-not-green grass stretches in every direction broken only by the giant mechanical bird-beak of the oil pumps as they dip, suck, dip, suck petroleum out of the veins of the earth. Mr. Import/Export's place is situated on a chunk of dry cracked earth best left to the wild hare and the prairie dog. Tumbleweeds and torn plastic bags scramble across the yard as if they are desperate to get away. This has to be my least favourite part of the city so far. If I had to live here, I feel like I'd never have another good idea again.

When we arrive Mr. Import/Export lets us in but fixes us with a cold stare. He has a sore throat he says. He had to go and get an antibiotic because he can't afford to be sick. He'll go to the bedroom and try to make us a sample but he isn't sure he'll be able to. Oh, a sore throat, I think. Poor baby. He hasn't turned on any music or anything, and so we flip on the television, just to fill the silence and give him some privacy while we sit there. Unfortunately, he has some satellite system that either isn't working properly or needs a code to turn it on. All we can get is one fuzzy analog channel where unidentified players bat a tennis ball back and forth. It would be great entertainment for a cat, perhaps, but doesn't do much for us.

After about forty-five minutes he emerges with a baggy that he hands to us while opening the door for us to leave. He doesn't even say goodbye, just shuts the door in our faces.

"That was weird," I say to Viviën when we get back in the car.

"He's a creep." She says out loud what we have likely both been thinking for some time but didn't want to admit. Now here we are driving across town with a sandwich baggie of sperm from someone we don't even like. Stranger than fiction, life is, I swear. What are we going to do with it? Is it even worth putting it in there at all? Maybe we should just throw it out the window. We think about this for some time, but in the end, the stuff is just too hard to come by that we can't bear to.

"Even sperm from a creep is better than no sperm at all." I quip, making up an adage that I'm pretty sure no one else has ever used before.

We are terribly annoyed and not in the mood to get into bed at all when we get back home. We love one another other tremendously, however, and we really want a family. So we get the job done, and I lie with the feet in the air for an hour before going off to a rehearsal for my play that a Calgary theatre company is mounting. It is about a woman who is out in her kayak and finds a floating head. She calls various authorities but no one wants to take responsibility for it. This systemic "not my department" response sends her into a giggling fit. Suddenly the police, who up until then were thoroughly convinced that there was nothing they could do, prick up their ears. Maybe this laughing woman (isn't it odd to laugh at mortality?) might have something to do with the crime. Just as water will always find the most direct route to rejoin its other molecules, suspicion once aroused will always find a target to fix upon. I wonder if my kids, once they get to an age where they could do so, will want to read my work. If they do, will they find it and me weird?

By now our trust in Mr. Import/Export is seriously eroded, and it seems pretty clear to us that his enthusiasm for our family plans have waned. We have to let him go.

## 23. bigdaddybear

While looking through a list of Calgary's gay organizations I come upon what sounds like the holy grail of sperm donation: the Calgary Gay Dads Association. I fire off a request to join, daydreaming of all the prospective donors we could meet, not to mention the dinner parties with good wine. Not that I have anything against lentils, hummus or herbal tea, and there's nothing wrong with a good potluck, but I'm looking forward to changing things up a bit. I get a message back in short order saying that the group (quite understandably) restricts its membership to people who are actually gay dads. Once I explain our plight, however, the kind web admin guy agrees to forward our request to their membership.

To our great excitement, we begin to get messages almost immediately. The first is from a fellow using the handle BigDaddyBear. He writes that he works in construction and is the father of three wonderful kids. He had the children with his former wife, with whom he split amicably when he came to terms with his feelings for men. He now has joint custody of his children. He lives down the street from his ex-wife and the children have rooms in both places. BigDaddyBear also shares with us that he has recently found and proposed to the man of his dreams.

I write back to him eagerly, congratulating him on being true to himself, arranging his family situation so well and finding love. I suggest that we meet in a funky brew pub in the downtown. He agrees, saying that he has been wanting to try that particular pub anyway. At the end of the message BigDaddyBear says he is really looking forward to our meeting, hopes we will hit it off and adds somewhat coyly that there is a twist.

"A twist, what does that mean, a twist?" asks Viviën.

I read his message to her and then say, "I don't know. A twist can be something good, right? Let's keep an open mind."

She nods. We both know that we are landlocked for the winter and our prospects are fairly limited. As long as the twist doesn't carry a prison sentence we're probably still interested.

When we arrive the pub is jammed. Viviën heads over to the bar to get us drinks and I try to find an elbow's width of room on one of the huge polished tables. The happy hour crowd just off the red mile is in full roar, and the music is louder than it really ought to be for detailed conversation. I have no idea how we will find him, and so I begin a text to prospective donor to ask if he has arrived when suddenly a mountain of a man is towering over me, blocking out all of the light. He is so massive that it is difficult to take him in at close range. It seems impossible that he could be a civilian. He must be an offensive tackle for the Stampeders, a professional wrestler or one of those modern-day strong men who flip cars and toss around tractor tires. He has a big bushy beard, which curls out from cherry red lips and does not hide his friendly smile and twinkling blue eyes. In fact he looks a bit like Santa. A virile Santa who works out. And takes steroids.

"I think we're looking for one another," he says and extends an enormous hand, the size and shape of a shovel blade. I brace for a bone cruncher, but his touch is gentle, and he turns the shake into a kind of lift and before I know it I am being propelled toward a place where we can sit down. I am of medium height, but standing up with my boots on my eyes are only level with the second button of his shirt. I can see why he picked the email handle BigDaddyBear. He has a presence that could be called commanding, and the human sea in front of us simply parts for him. Suddenly we have a table all to ourselves in a corner away from the largest of the loudspeakers. I see Viviën surfing the wave of office workers with icy drafts in hand.

The three of us make our introductions. There is a round of pleasant, light conversation about construction (an interest that he and Viviën have in common), about children (which he has and we would like to have) and about brew pubs (because we are sitting in one and because BigDaddyBear plans to open one). We have all finished two-thirds of a beer and the conversation has warmed to the point where I feel it is a good moment to start talking about the donation, but BigDaddyBear beats me to the punch.

"I know you came here tonight thinking that I would be your donor, but…" Here he pauses and rubs his massive hands together. Our heads snap up. A "but," while not entirely a novelty at this stage, is still a bit of a blow to the solar plexus. "I have something else in mind," he says. Ah yes. This must be the "twist" that he mentioned in his email.

It is a testament to just how much we want a family that neither Viviën nor I jump up and run screaming into the night. Instead we hear him out. It seems that he is entirely happy with his lot in life. He has fathered, fed, burped and changed three babies. It has been one of the best experiences of his life but he doesn't have any desire to be a donor. What he is really interested in is setting us up with his new partner, who, it seems, has not had the experience of fatherhood and would benefit hugely from this opportunity. He beams at us with good humour but we can't help but wonder why the fellow didn't write to us himself. And for that matter, why isn't he here?

BigDaddyBear tells us that his lover is a very sensitive soul with a big heart. He is a gifted chef who dreams of opening his own restaurant. Since he and BigDaddyBear have been together, he has had a chance to interact with the kids, and he has seen just how much happiness children bring to your life. But, BigDaddyBear does not want to have more children since his own are now entering their teens. So when he saw our message a light bulb went off and he convinced his lover to meet up with us after his shift at a nearby restaurant. As if on cue, the young man shows up. And young is the best word to describe him. This provokes a whole range of unnameable emotions in me, and I can see Viviën's eyes widen as she takes him in. He is wearing a baseball hat, worn jeans and a hoodie, and if there had been someone on the door asking for identification he would certainly have been carded. He is also skinny and pale and has large liquid brown puppy dog eyes. I note the hunched shoulders of a kid who expects a kick or a blow, be it real or metaphorical, to come at some point from the outside world. My immediate thought is that I want to give this boy a bowl of soup, a pep talk and a hug, not ask him to father our children.

Nonetheless he sits down, and we find out he is actually in his early twenties, not a teenager. He is likeable, and by the time he's downed his second draft, we have heard his tragic life story. He grew up with his mother in a mud lot in a fifth wheel trailer on Vancouver Island. His father was abusive — he saw his mom beaten in front of him for most of his childhood. It was a logging town with one grocery store and nothing to do. He turned to drugs pretty heavily and pretty early for solace.

His description does not coincide with the view that most people have of Vancouver Island, which normally conjures up old-growth forests, organic farms and communal living. But then there is the interior. And the picture he describes rings true. A rural community with everyone scratching a living from the forest (in my case it was the fishery). In places like that there are no women's shelters, no teen drop-in centres. Where I grew up there was nowhere to run to either. Now into my third beer, this kid is tearing me up with his story. "Finally the asshole left, but Ma found another one even worse. One night I had enough, stepped in the middle. He kicked my ass basically but I got my licks in. Ma gave me the money she had and I left. I figured I would go to Van, but the city ate me alive. No work to be had. All the shelters were full and skid row is a total shitshow. I knew I had to get out. Everyone was saying that in Calgary you could get work so I jumped the bus. That very same night I met my saviour," he says, hooking a thumb with nails bitten down to the quick at BigDaddyBear.

"Best night of my life," says BigDaddyBear.

"I had seven bucks in my pocket," the kid laughs, "not even enough to buy my own pack of smokes."

"We hit it off right away," says BigDaddyBear.

"He gave me a place to stay..."

"We have a lot in common, he's an old soul."

"And I never left."

"And now we're going to be married."

"Whatever you say."

"And we're going to open a restaurant together. He is a very talented chef."

"Don't call me a chef. I wash dishes for a living."

"For now, but I'm thinking of the future."

"I like washing dishes."

While these two seem to have different narratives about both their past and their future, this is of little concern to us. Most couples do. In fact, don't we all pretty much live in our own stories and dance the happy dance when they happen to converge with the stories of those we love?

What is worrying is that the desire for the kid to be a donor seems to be coming entirely from BigDaddyBear. The kid is apathetic about the idea at best. He is very sweet and is clearly enjoying talking to us. But he seems so newly sprung from his own broken family that the furthest thing from his mind is helping someone start their own. When we tell him the kind of arrangement we have in mind, especially the part about the donor being known to the child at some future date, he looks doubtful.

"I guess I wouldn't mind if the kid wanted to track me down. I don't know. I wouldn't say no if you're hell bent on it. I did a lot of drugs, though. Not now, before. Would that give them, like, defects? I don't know anything about that shit. Would that affect a kid? I'm just being honest, you know. I got my life on track now, but you know. The island. Nothing to do. You blaze, you huff, whatever. I just want you to know that. I mean I would totally give you nice girls some ghiz if you want it, but I don't want to, like, vouch for it. If something bad happens."

Although it is very unlikely that any kind of donation will come out of this evening's meeting, we laugh, chat, drink another beer and enjoy the company of two interesting people we would not otherwise have met. As we say goodnight, they promise to invite us to their next big dinner party.

## 24. contemplating anonymity

After being emotionally curb-stomped by near strangers and spending the better part of an hour each morning fielding emails from raging megalomaniacs who want to conquer North America through prodigious mail order distribution of their sperm, the idea of an anonymous donor, which at first we dismissed out of hand, starts to gain some traction.

An anonymous sperm donor wasn't what we wanted in the beginning, and all of our objections about that still stand. It seemed like a bit of a missed opportunity to have an anonymous donor when you could offer a child another adult who could be an important figure in their life. In an ideal world we also want to give them the opportunity to form a relationship with their biological father. Most importantly, we have Viviën's experience as an adopted child who grew up wondering about her origins. We want to give our children the opportunity to satisfy their natural curiosity about their roots.

Another consideration is the conception itself. We would rather have this spark, this moment of origin of our baby, take place during an intimate moment and be born of an act of love, not offload it to a sterile doctor's office. All of these feelings are still with us, but we have put our hopes and dreams in the hands of strangers and that has not worked out. We spent a year courting sperm donors, and their decisions and actions have impacted us hugely.

"I'm sorry Blanche Dubois, it may be here that we part ways," I mutter, as I pick up and leaf through the sperm donor catalogue that we received in the mail after an initial inquiry at the fertility clinic. I am losing my taste for letting other people's schedules have such an impact on our lives. I dog ear a page and pass it to Viviën.

"What about him?"

"Did you read the hobbies?" asks Viviën, "computer games, linex and comic books?"

"Okay, how about him?"

"Five foot one?"

Here we go with the height thing again. It is astounding, but there are almost no voluntary sperm donors over five foot five, and the few that are there are maxed out. Thankfully, in Canada there is a maximum number of children that can be created from any one anonymous sperm donor. This is to minimize the chances of people who are biologically related to one another meeting and pairing up down the road. And also to avoid creating artificially high numbers of people from the same gene pool. Of the fifty or so donor profiles, only three are over six feet, and they are either at or approaching their number of donations, while the shorter donors remain available.

Again, I wonder why this is so. Are we really so motivated by physical traits? Is this the primitive part of the brain kicking in and trying to choose the largest, strongest mate to ensure the survival of our young? You must understand that when I say "we," I don't just mean lesbian and other women seeking sperm. The preference for height also appears to be a major motivator for women who select their mate and breed the standard way. Could this be why human beings are getting taller and taller every year? I thought it was the milk. Or, more sinisterly, the growth hormones in the milk … but anyway, those poor short men. Suddenly I feel really bad for them. I thought it was bad for me trying to find a date in rural Nova Scotia; maybe they had an even tougher time. Perhaps the only chance that men of shorter stature have to spread their genetic material is via this very catalogue. Maybe we should give them a chance. I don't want to be having the thoughts I'm having right now but it seems impossible to turn the monkey brain off.

"Okay, what about him?" I ask, pointing out a profile of a man with Caribbean ancestry.

"A dark guy would be okay for you," she says. "I don't want it for me though."

"But we wanted to have the same donor for both. And Mr. Import/ Export was black," I argue.

"I know, but he was live and he was the only chance we had. I didn't feel like I had a choice. If we are going to choose out of a catalogue, I don't want a dark guy."

"I don't understand. Why not?"

"It just doesn't feel right."

You can't argue with feelings, so we move on. Poring over the fine print of the catalogue, I read something disturbing. It says that if you want to have a donor who is of a different ethnic background than you, you need to go for counselling. Bizarre! Does that mean they think that straight interracial couples need counselling too?

The politics of regulating genetic material, if you start looking into them, are deeply conflicted. In Canada, unlike the United States, a donor cannot profit monetarily from donating any genetic material. The legislation seems well intentioned as it wants to protect those who find themselves in difficult circumstances from harvesting and selling off their own body parts. This might seem like science fiction, but as I recently discovered while doing research on this topic for a play, this nightmarish scenario is all too real. There are several grisly international markets where you can buy anything from a kidney to a cornea from a living donor. Reputedly these donors sell their body parts of their own free will, but free will is a wiggly concept when it is mixed on the open market with savage capitalism. Yes, free will breaks down when buyers cross borders from developed to developing nations (although I hate to reinforce that horrible binary). What if you lived in poverty and the sale of a kidney could buy your child an education that she would not otherwise have? What if that education meant that she had a chance at a job or a career, at a life beyond mere subsistence? You might not live as long, but you have purchased your child's ticket out. What makes sense from one perspective is, from another angle, a horrific prospect. Of course the flow of body parts follows the lines of power and privilege, and it pushes at the uneasy boundary between the free market and human rights.

So I fully support the Canadian position that any transaction of biological material be motivated by altruism and hence operate under what is called the "gift economy." This usually means that you donate an egg to your sister who is infertile to help her have a baby. Or that your healthy brother gives you a kidney that will save you from a life chained to a dialysis machine. We can all understand the logic there. Most of us, if you come right down to it, would open ourselves up at the seam from head to toe and offer up any part we have to save the ones we love. When it comes to sperm, however, the idea of the gift economy doesn't quite jive. First of all, unlike some donations, this one is pretty much free from physical pain and health risks. Yet without compensation very few men turn up at the clinic to donate their sperm in the spirit of altruism. You can't ask someone who is biologically related to you to be your sperm donor for obvious reasons, and so here we can feel the ribbon on this bright package of the gift economy stretch and strain.

In the U.S., on the other hand, you can buy eggs or sperm or both at an increasingly proliferating number of clinics, and the free market surrounding reproductive material has created a kind of wild west mentality. So you have little Yale sperms and little Princeton ova sell for thousands or hundreds of thousands of dollars — the inflated worth above that of other healthy genetic material based on a grim calculus of wealth, status, class and privilege with no grounding whatsoever in science.

A brief glance through the pages of history debunks the notion that greatness is passed on genetically. I believe fervently that a bright flame can emerge from any corner of the earth, that each and every human, no matter what conditions they might be born into, can light its wick. Quite without regard to my lofty ideals, however, the trade in Ivy League eggs and sperm goes at a brisk pace. This is in line with the hard facts of life for a student in urban centres in the States: if you want to get into one of the elite schools you'd better go to the right high school. To get in there you would have needed to attend one of a select number of grade schools, which in term only look at students who have attended X, Y and Z preschools. Parents who want to get their kid into one of those preschools better be prepared to drop some money on a hefty tuition fee and put them on a waiting list for five years prior to attending. Yes, this means putting your kids on a waiting list for kindergarten before they even exist.

That must be some pretty special colouring. Some pretty elite ABCs. We're talking networking sessions between power naps and organic gluten free bites that we won't deign to call cookies. The logical extension of these ways of paying for the best possible start in life for your children is, perhaps in some cases, buying genetic material that is "superior" to your own.

*You know I'm not saying you're stupid, honey. I'm just saying that if we really want junior to succeed, then we should do the right thing for him and get sperm with higher grades in math.*

*Well your eggs aren't exactly Stanford material either, sweetie. Maybe you should drop that People Magazine and pick up the Huffington Post.*

Then you have a lot of activity swarming on the margins of the law. Some Canadians leave the country to buy sperm because they know that if the donor is not a Canadian citizen, it is unlikely he will emerge in future to claim parental rights. While attending the University of Calgary, I remember seeing advertisements in the student paper offering qualified donors a free trip to Australia as long as they were willing to trade a sperm donation for a few days of sand and surf. Many Canadians frustrated by the government's regulations around donor sperm and eggs travel to the Czech Republic, where clinics will put you up for a week during your ovulation window and drench you in sperm every few hours. Unlike our own clinics, which give stern warnings not to get your hopes up and advise you to set aside a year and a good chunk of your life savings just to "try" getting pregnant, the Czech clinics offer a money-back guarantee.

Unlike in Canada, where the laws pretty much guarantee that anyone who offers you an egg donation will be an invested donor (a sister or a friend, for example), French law prohibits this type of altruistically motivated donation. The current practice, then, for an infertile French woman who is capable of carrying a child and has a willing known donor is to travel to Belgium, where the practice is permitted. The fact that Canadian law prohibits paying men for sperm donation (other than to compensate them for the hour that they might miss work) means that not as many men donate here as they do in countries like Sweden and Denmark, where sperm donation is a relatively well-compensated favourite side job of university students. In fact the Scandinavian countries give so many donations that you picture the earth being soon populated with little blonde Swedes and Danes. Whenever the law impinges upon or tries to limit the power of the human body, it tends to rear up in its tracks like a skittish pony.

We discover that there is only one fertility clinic in the country that allows couples to do home insemination. This clinic is in Ontario. The sperm bank it deals with helpfully sent us a list of profiles to choose from. With a prescription from our doctor we can purchase a sperm sample from them that will be cleaned, frozen, packed in dry ice and FedExed to our door.

After talking through all of this again, we decide that all of our original objections to an anonymous donor still stand. We still think looking for someone to be our donor and attempting to conceive children on our own is the best option for us, but Operation Spermination is being impeded by geography. For this reason we decide to pack up house in Calgary. I am teaching a field school in Vienna, after which we plan to visit family and friends in Holland. We'll then spend the balance of the summer on Bowen Island, B.C. This is a little island off the coast of Vancouver where we spent some time a couple of years back and fell in love with. We have had queries from a couple of potential donors in Vancouver, and we're thinking that perhaps we might have more luck finding a like-minded fellow on the west coast. The island has beaches and forest and fresh air, and very importantly, it is close enough to hop the ferry over to the mainland when needed.

## 25. leaning dangerously from a fourth-storey window in Vienna

There are moments in the journey of life when you have to ask yourself how you got so far away from the goal you thought you were pursuing, and this could be one of those moments. Right now the biggest thing on my mind is how we can have a baby. How will we get pregnant? Where will we find the right donor and how will we arrange all of the delicate events in the right order to nudge this very much desired little being into the world? Why then, do I find myself standing on a radiator and leaning dangerously out of a fourth-storey window of a mouldering pension near the opera house in Vienna trying to catch a wifi signal with my laptop?

There is likely a larger answer that might involve soul searching and an exhaustive study of the gypsy-like propensity for movement that has traced my life since I left home at seventeen. But, I'll stick to the short answer here. I designed and am piloting a field study program for my theatre and creative writing students that takes place at a theatre festival in Austria. I am waiting for all of them to arrive for the two weeks we'll spend here together studying. I always bemoan the fact that I often end up teaching theatre to students who are either disinclined or who don't have enough time to go and see live theatre. For them, the plays exist only as a flat blueprint on a page, and it is left to me to try and animate them. Haul the character, set, period, the entire flavour of a piece up out of the book and into the room. I love to do it and often, I think, succeed, but I know how much more powerful dramatic works are if you can see them live. The starting point for this field study is that I have always worked best and with the most creative fire when I am under the influence of, or inspired by, another writer's or troupe's work. Of course, as a writer, there is a fair amount of sitting alone in my room and putting the proverbial nose to the figurative grindstone. But there is really nothing like those dizzying first moment when you walk out of a theatre where you have just been moved. You have seen something you never witnessed before, and it is causing you to fire on all pistons. Everything seems possible and you can see your next masterpiece hanging in the air.

I want to give my students — developing writers, some new and some well on their way — this experience. To this end I devised a syllabus based on the works appearing at Vienna's avant-garde festival of international theatre called Weiner Festwochen. We study and discuss a series of plays that we see together. The students also work on their own writing projects while they are immersed in the creative ambiance of the festival. We are all staying at a very affordable pension (midway between a hostel and a hotel) right in the heart of the city. From here I could throw a baseball and hit three or four theatres, two museums and countless number of art galleries. Not that I would. It would probably be frowned upon. We are so close to the opera house that I can hear the top notes of the soprano as she blows it out at the end of *Salome.*

This well-thought-out plan, to my mind, has the potential to create pretty much an ideal teaching/learning environment. Nevertheless, I still have a class of university-age students arriving via overseas flights and unfamiliar public transit routes to check into this mostly darkened pension sometime this evening and in the wee hours of the morning. The group has varying degrees of experience in travel; some are intent on study, some on exploring Europe and some on partying. And most are intent on striking a balance between all three under my charge for the completion of two full courses. I heard horror stories from other professors who have run these field schools about how they sometimes come back a student short. Someone loses it and bolts. One student eloped on him, my colleague told me. I remember swallowing hard. Of course they are adults and can make their own decisions but if at all possible I'd like to come back with the same number of students that I left Calgary with. Also, I am not sure how much experimental theatre or avant-garde art of any sort they will have seen. My syllabus features no *Oklahoma*, no *Cats*. Not even the dignified death of a hardworking salesman. The first play that I will take them to see is a sprawling nine-hour epic by Quebec's consummate postmodern showman Robert Lepage, and due to the vagaries of scheduling we will have to see this tomorrow on the first day of the course while they are still jetlagged. Oh well, nothing like leaping in with both feet. If nothing else, this will be an experience they won't soon forget.

Despite all of this going through my mind, there is still a part of me that is always focused on our main project. We need to spend the summer in Vancouver or surrounding area so that we can find a donor, so that we can start a family. It is quite difficult to find any kind of a summer rental on Bowen Island , and so I am combing through the classified section of the little local paper on the smallest coastal island. The internet signal is weak and broadcast from the pension office, which is closed. And that is why I am, right now, in the middle of the night, leaning dangerously out of a fourth storey window in a moldering pension.

## 26. hitchhiker to the candy store

Ever since we visited Bowen Island a few years ago, we have been dreaming of eventually creating a life out there. Unlike most of the Gulf Islands, which are closer to Vancouver Island, this one is just off the mainland. You can actually see the lights of the West End, and if traffic and ferry schedules cooperate you can be in downtown Vancouver in under an hour. Yet Bowen still maintains that quirky west coast island feeling left over from the hippy days when those tired of the "rat race" cashed in their chips and went out to the islands to build houses out of driftwood and grow organic vegetables. Driving along, we were shocked to see a boy of eight or nine stick out his thumb to hitch a ride. When we pulled over he explained that he needed a lift to the candy store.

"Sure, we can give you a ride. I just want to know, though, is it okay with your folks if you hitchhike?

"Of course," he laughed. "Not on the mainland," he says, shading the word with a bit of danger, "but kids hitch all the time out here on the island."

This incident lodged itself in my mind. As did the vast tracks of untouched Pacific rainforest, the countless coves and beaches and the one very quiet ring road that circles most of the island. It seemed to be a perfect place for a kid. You could play outside for hours at a time. Swim from rafts, catch fish, ride bikes and climb rocks. All the good kid stuff.

Bowen is a place where teachers are eager, where they compete to come and teach grade one in the public school system. I can imagine children out there still being allowed to run wild in the woods, bike to their friends' places and wake up every summer morning shouldering the decision of which swimming beach to meet their friends at. Should they build a raft or catch some crabs?

As we rounded the corner, the boy, who said his name was Zack, suddenly yelled: "Stop! Stop right here. This is the best corner for blackberries!"

We pulld over and he grabed them by the handful, stuffing them in his mouth and staining his hands.

"Come on, get some," he beckoned us, and we jumped out and picked as many berries as we could, piling them in the front of our t-shirts. We munched them the rest of the way down the hill. Zack was right, that was the best corner for blackberries. We arrived at the cove and he got out.

"Who needs candy when you have blackberrries, eh, Zack?"

"I do!" he said and with a wave disappeared around the corner.

That cinched it. Bowen Island is perhaps the last place on earth where a nine-year-old can safely hitch to the candy store. If we have kids, we have to take them there. That said, that seeming paradise is no longer the wide-open hippie haven it was when many of the folks built the self-starter log homes, eccentric dome houses and panabodes, which are ready made wooden house kits popular in the 1970s that make up the bulk of the houses on the island. Since then there has been a major real estate spike and a boom of construction. Vancouver is now one of the most expensive cities in the world and this is turning the island into a bedroom community for commuters. This is changing its flavour from a retreat for hippies and artists to a very pricey place to live. Even the most humble cottage now costs half a million. Yes, half a million. This seems nutty to me, hailing as I do from the Maritimes, where if a house costs that much we expect one of the members of the royal family to have stayed there or have at least stopped there to take a leak.

Bowen Island's bucolic seaside lifestyle has become complicated. The main topics on the town web forum seem to be: 1. Development 2. How to stop it. This paradigm is not particular to this island, however. It seems that folks everywhere, after finding their paradise, want to pull up the drawbridge on the moat right after they arrive. Having gained access to paradise themselves, folks often become abruptly reluctant to share it.

Thus, it is very tough to find a reasonably priced long-term rental on the island. There is no campground either. I exchange some emails with a woman who is putting her house on the market. She says we can rent it, but we'd have to leave at short notice if she sells it. This suits us fine, and I send her a deposit. A few weeks before we are to arrive, unfortunately (for us) but fortunately (for her), she does, indeed, sell her house, leaving us temporarily homeless.

From my nest atop the perch in my pension room in Vienna I comb the online classifieds. I finally find a self-contained, two-bedroom suite on the main floor of a house right on the ocean. We'd rather rent a whole house, but the advertisement promises privacy, a separate entrance and an amazing view. I contact the owners and write several desperate emails negotiating for the presence of our model citizen dog as the original advertisement said no pets preferred. I extol his virtue and pledge my life on his cleanliness and sociability. I follow this with a wire transfer of two months' rent plus a damage deposit chaser, and this is enough to secure the apartment for us. At least now we'll have a place to land when we get there.

## 27. separating the nuts

A few weeks later we arrive on the island, having caught the last ferry from Horseshoe Bay. Before that we had an intercontinental flight with a nasty layover in Heathrow. We spent the last few hours in the city getting the basic things we need to set up. In tow, we have a friend of Viviën's from Holland, who will be visiting us for a week or so. Before any of us can sleep we'll have to unwrap sheets and make up beds.

I have been communicating with the woman who owns the house

and am expecting to have a quick hello tonight, pick up a key and meet with her again in the morning. She, however, is not at home when we arrive. And so instead of her, we get her husband. He is a German fellow that we'll call Wolfgang, who has either very poor social skills or a severe case of paranoia. I just wish she had given us a heads-up. When we arrive he produces a standard short-term lease agreement, which we read and sign within three minutes. But then he proceeds to pore over it for an hour and a half as if it contains the answer to the riddles of the sphinx, the Rosetta stone and the Caramilk secret rolled into one.

We want to start off on the right foot. We will be living downstairs from these folks for at least a few months, but we are so tired. All we want to do is get clean and sleep. Finally, I tell him thank you but we're very tired and ask if we can just get a key for now and handle the rest in the morning.

"A key." He repeats my words in a flat tone, as if I might have some sinister motive.

"Yes, a key. Can we have a key for the suite, so that if we go out we can lock it?" A glimmer of light dawns somewhere and he pats his pockets. I think we are home free but then I make the mistake, since I am standing near the door, of reaching over and trying the handle to see if it is a twist lock or a keyed lock.

It is sticky and lets out a loud squeak. Rather than give us a key, Wolfgang becomes fascinated by the stickiness of the locking mechanism and decides to take the whole thing apart there and then. I am not sure whether to cry or scream. We have been driving for twenty hours, and aside from a brief stopover with friends in Calgary, we've been on the road for a month. Now he has the door off the hinges. Why won't this man just go away? Another torturous half hour goes by while he shows us around the suite. Here's how the windows work: they go up and down. A stove, yes, off and on. The fridge, open and shut. There goes the little light. Excellent, thank you. In addition to being overly invested in minute details, he is also weirdly concerned with bathroom functions. He spends a good twenty minutes in there explaining pretty basic matters of drainage and asking us how often we go to the bathroom, and I begin to wonder if he has some kind of weird fetish. Even after he gives me the practical explanation of his concern for his newly installed above-ground septic tank, his single-minded devotion to the topic of body fluids is still unsettling.

Okay we might have to find somewhere else to stay tomorrow if he is going to be a problem, but tonight we just need to sleep. I take his elbow firmly but gently and escort him to the door, which is still only provisionally attached to the frame. He makes a grab for it, but I keep on steering until he is around the corner and up the stairs. "We'll manage. Goodnight!" I come back inside and switch off the lights just to make sure he gets the message.

Vivien and I and her friend all stare at each other until we hear him continue up his stairs and into his part of the house. We breathe a sigh of relief and settle in for the night. For the rest of our time here, it turns out to be hard to avoid Wolfgang, despite his continual assertions that he is "busy, so busy" and that he "can't stop to talk, he has too much to do." He still obstructs our path and subjects us to fifteen-minute monologues on the merits of one type of cleaning fluid over another. We try to read a book on the deck of the suite and he's up on the second floor deck pretending to water the plants and peeking down through the planks. We are walking from the shower in a towel and he just happens to need to cross in front of the window on his way to the storage room. We go up the driveway to walk to the beach and there he is with his ancient VW mercilessly torn apart, elbow deep in grease with buckets of nuts and bolts spread around, and he is standing with a magnet.

"What you doing, Wolfgang?" I make the mistake of asking.

"Separating the stainless steel nuts from the regular ones," he replies. "But I can't talk, I have too much to do."

I leave him there, separating his nuts, and resolve to simply duck him as much as possible in future. But this proves difficult as he doesn't work and never goes anywhere, and this means we pretty much run into him every time we leave or come back home. This is a bummer because he isn't just an odd duck who keeps to himself. No, Wolfgang is zealously devoted to bathroom habits. His, ours and those of our guests, who, unfortunately, are treated to a speech on this topic. One day he even insists on giving a "tour" of his custom-made above-ground septic tank. *Be still my beating heart!*

Despite our repeated assurances that have completely uninteresting and average bathroom habits, Wolfgang takes to counting how many times we flush the toilet. If he catches my eye on my way out, he gives me his count by holding up his fingers through the window. Even though I keep asking him to respect our privacy, he finds excuses to tinker around tightening a screw on our deck or fiddling around with the garden hose at the side of the house. Even though I ask him nicely many times there doesn't seem to be any way of getting him to leave us alone. If we have people over, he just walks up to them and starts talking about plumbing. I actually catch him in the act of asking one of our guests if he's ever peed in the woods and if he *likes* to pee in the woods. Wolfgang is singlehandedly dampening my enthusiasm for this beautiful place and the breathtaking view.

## 28. make the call

We haven't managed to get a cell phone that works properly on the island. We bought a temporary cell phone and a plan, but it goes out of range somewhere in the Georgia Strait about the mid-way point between the island and the mainland, despite the assurances of the teen sales agent in the mall in North Vancouver, who told us we'd totally get a gnarly signal all over the island. Our signal is slightly less than gnarly, and by now I've learned to read my body enough to know that I'll be ovulating in a day or so. Our suitcases are in a pile in the corner, and we don't yet have groceries, but all of that will have to wait because we need sperm.

We don't want to let another month go by while we get settled. Even the extra day or so it will take to get a decent cell phone could mean missing my window of ovulation and we'll have to wait another month. For any other phone call I would likely just ask to use the phone of the people we are renting from, but given the bizarre peccadillos of the fellow we are renting from I really doubt that I could carry on a comprehensible conversation with our newest potential donor with Wolfgang in earshot.

We'll have to call him from somewhere else. A payphone, Viviën suggests but I don't even know if there is a payphone on the island. We set out to find one and are chagrined to discover that the island's only pay phone is within earshot of the outdoor patio of the only bar in town. This is less than ideal and there is yet another challenge. This island seems to have a high concentration of eccentrics, and one of them believes that she owns or is at least the protector of the pay phone. She isn't using it, but she isn't quite *not* using it either. When I ask her directly she says that she is waiting for a call. I ask if I can make one quick call. "But how will I know," she says, "if my call comes while you are on there?" I see her eyes are whirling and wild. Best not to try reasoning with her.

I want Viviën to be the one to call him, but she, likely tired from the trip and maybe just tired of the steeplechase in pursuit of sperm, doesn't want to. This ticks me off because it is in direct violation of our agreement that we would do the negotiation for one another. I remind her of this and she reluctantly agrees. We dig out a quarter from the ashtray and I give her the number. She tries it several times. She comes back to the truck. Maybe it's the phone or maybe it's the number, but for whatever reason she can't get a connection. I have become a grumpy little shrew by this time and snatch the quarter, slam the truck door and stomp over to the phone. This time, for whatever reason, the number rings through fine, and our potential new donor, who we know only by his email username, picks up instantly. I am not quite ready for this, still stewing as I am in my little moment, but this is such an important call that I recover fast. Our potential donor is in town at the moment, he is free and available to meet us the following day.

Viviën must be shocked, sitting in a truck, to see a smile suddenly spread across my face. It is a brief conversation but I like the sound of his voice. I skip back to the truck nodding to the lady protector of the phone that she can have her spot back.

"He's in town! He's game! He says he can meet us tomorrow!"

## 29. *a walk in the park*

As we have continued our dating process, the initial meeting with a potential donor has devolved from a dinner out, to a latte at Starbucks, to a coffee at Tim Hortons, to the super-efficient meeting we have arranged with our new potential donor: a walk in the park with the dog. Experience has taught us to leave ourselves an exit route and to invest less at the outset. This, I suppose, is a way of protecting ourselves from getting our hopes up too high. We walk around False Creek, a beautiful park that has been created over what used to be an industrial wasteland in downtown Vancouver.

Our new potential donor makes a good first impression. He has a direct, warm gaze, asks good questions and seems at ease in his body. He is informed, progressive and on the whole really comfortable with the idea of helping us start a family. He likes dogs. Bonus. Does volunteer work with kids in the great outdoors. Double bonus. As we stroll along the sea wall, the light conversation ranges from our mutual backgrounds and paths of study, then to his travels and our renovation projects. So far so good, but by now my antennae have become quite used to searching for early warning signs that the boat might capsize. These include, but aren't limited to, raging egomaniacs, men who are looking for sugarmamas, sperminators (men who want to populate the earth with their progeny indiscriminately) and men who would really rather have children of their own. I gradually relax as he tells us about his life and none of these flags goes up. He isn't in a relationship at the moment and so isn't sure if he'll end up having children of his own, but if he does he is open to and likes the idea of those children possibly having a relationship with our kids. He likes the idea of being known to the children as their biodad at some future point.

We find our way to a place to sit on an outdoor terrace for a coffee and this too goes well. We must pass muster for him too, because we agree to try when my next ovulation hits.

## 30. to the Sylvia on rollerblades

Our new donor glides along the seawall on rollerblades to the Sylvia Hotel in the early summer sunshine. I know this because I am perched in the window of the topmost corner of the building, watching for his approach. He is going to give us a sample of his sperm so that my wife can try and get me pregnant. This is really going to happen. As I see him approaching, I note that he's wearing linen. I can tell because linen has a special way of catching the air and flapping in the wind. The light bounces off his wheels. He could be Hermes, messenger to the gods with wings on his feet. When we asked him why he wanted to be a donor, he said this was just such a simple thing for him to do and it could make such a big difference to a couple who couldn't otherwise have a child. It just made sense to him to help out.

*Hey, Blanche, what do you know? We've found him. The last kindly stranger in the Modern World.*

I know I shouldn't inflate him to hero status as doing that to any mortal, no matter what they have done for you, is usually trouble. Better to keep him human. Better for us, for him, for the children that could result. However, I feel a kind of magic about the whole situation. Usually attempting to make things "perfect" brings about counterintuitive results. This time, though, we might have cheated fate.

I have a feeling that Vancouver — this city where I found my footing as a writer and as a young woman — is lucky for me. Maybe here it will work out. The Sylvia was the first place I stayed when I arrived on the west coast, green and wide-eyed from Nova Scotia. Just laying eyes on that neon sign with its classic "S" and the ivy-covered walls causes a deep sense of peace to seep up out of the cracked concrete all around me. The Sylvia caught me when I first landed, and it is the hotel I have always aspired to hole up in if ever I were to become the urban hermit of moderate means afforded to a doyenne of Canadian playwriting. Now that the path of my life is altering, this place still carries magic for me. If we stay here tonight, I think we can make a baby.

There are elements of practicality as well to the decision. We want things to be as convenient as possible for our donor and so staying on the mainland makes sense. We are, it is important to remember, asking someone to come into an unfamiliar environment and masturbate into a cup on our behalf, and we really can't expect that person to manage this in a car or a public washroom. Nor do we want to pick up the sperm from him and speed back to the ferry line, trying to keep it warm. If the little swimmers lose their mojo, then all of that fuss could be for nothing and we'd have to wait another month. But mostly I knew that it had to be the Sylvia because of the way I feel when I am here. They have somehow distilled what I love about Vancouver and dispense it with the room key when you sign in. Oh yes, and they give biscuits and greetings to your dog. This is important because I believe that once you extend your family unit to include a furry creature, you can't just abandon them when you go off on vacation. Rockit is always greeted with ear scratches and compliments, which puts him in an excellent mood. He gets a pronounced air of wounded dignity when someone insinuates he might be a bother. *What, me? I wouldn't dream of peeing on the carpets. What are we here, barbarians? Chew the moulding? Are you insane? Do you know how hard that stuff is to replace?* Whenever hysterical anti-dog people make wide circles around him, pointing their fingers at him, he only inclines his head sagely as if sorry for them. *How rude,* he seems to say, extending his front paws and stretching himself out with a yawn. *Your bitch should have brought you up with better manners.*

When we arrived the handsome young gay man on the front desk gave us a big wide smile and an upgrade, slipping us the keys to the top corner room with the windows right on English Bay while only charging us the normal rate. The sun was shining, bouncing off the water, and the boats were bobbing like brightly painted toys. The whole day seemed to be flowing along as if stage managed by a creative genius with attention to detail.

Then, for reasons I don't understand, I panicked. Maybe it was the shock of finally getting down to business after all of the waiting and planning, but my skull lit up like a pinball machine on tilt. I suddenly couldn't remember whether we made it absolutely clear that he would be putting his sperm into a cup and not into me. I mean we used the term donor and we discussed all the pertinent details about the children, that he wouldn't have any responsibilities toward them, and so on. But I was suddenly not entirely sure that he somehow couldn't have misconstrued what we wanted and that he might be coming here intending to give what is referred to as a natural donation, in other words to have intercourse. Some people do arrange things this way, but we definitely do not want this.

A misunderstanding at this stage of the game would be unbearable. On top of that, I realized that despite all the time we have spent in pursuit of sperm, and all the days and hours of planning we have spent on this, now that we have another willing donor, we haven't even brought any sort of receptacle for him to put the sperm into. And we don't have time to run out and buy anything. There is a tiny glass cup, the size of a shot glass, but I wasn't sure it was sanitized, whether the size might be requiring a bit too much accuracy, or how we would get it out of there afterward. The upshot of all this was that I begged Viviën to call him and ask him to bring some kind of flask along. She called him and he was excellent. He said he knew of just the thing: a small plastic sterile container of the right size. He is going to rollerblade over from his place along the sea wall and he will stop at the pharmacy on the way and pick one up. He also asked us if we want him to come by in the morning as well because he's read that success rates are higher when you make two attempts. Wow, he's perfect, I thought again.

Our donor, thankfully, isn't nervous when he arrives, or he's doing his best to cover it up, just like we are. We have the room tidy, and when I see him coming I flick the TV on, looking for some music to break the silence. I remember reading that in sperm clinics they have some "visual aids" to help the donors. Of course we have no such thing. I did consider this aspect, but I couldn't picture myself buying a girlie magazine. And I certainly wouldn't presume to know whether such a thing would help or hinder his process. I also couldn't see myself handing it over to him. I hoped that if he needed anything of this sort, he would bring it himself.

We chat for a moment or two and then Viviën and I leave to go for a quick walk on the beach with the dog. Our donor has our cell phone number, and so he can text us when he's finished. This text message will go on record as the most eagerly anticipated digital message we've ever received. As we ride the creaky elevator back up to our room, her eyes are dancing at the thought of what we are about to do. When we get back he takes a quick moment to scratch the dog's ears and then says: "It's on the counter in the bathroom, so I'll leave you to it." And he leaves without further small talk, which is very considerate. It would be hard to sit down and make polite conversation all the time worrying that our sperm—that is to say his sperm — is getting cold. That would be awkward, and after all this time, we're anxious to get this show on the road.

With the late afternoon sun bouncing off English Bay, in the upper-most corner of the Sylvia Hotel we go about the joyful business of (hopefully) starting our family. Afterward, Viviën helps me elevate my legs on a pile of pillows and I lie there upside down for likely far longer than is necessary. I gaze out over the flapping sails thinking welcoming baby thoughts and crossing my fingers. Somehow I just know that this time it will work. Maybe it's wishful thinking, but somehow I am sure that I can feel a baby immediately take root.

## 31. letters to possible creatures (dear baby to be)

After the upside down business, I sit down and write this, the first of several letters addressed to children we might have.

*Dear Baby To Be,*

*Right now, if all the documentaries I have watched about you are accurate, you are invisible to the naked eye. You are a couple of cells loaded with potential that might or might not meet one another for coffee. Of course you might also miss the appointment. You. An amazing chemical reaction. Right now a diminutive bundle of cells someplace inside me that might stick around and make a cozy spot. Make me heavy like a pear... change the course of my life. Teach me everything about my own folly worth knowing... I hope. I wish. I am wishing, right now for you to be settling in and going through the mind-rocking chemical cell-splitting fission type metamorphoses that you need to ... to grow into a precious little pollywog. Then a preternaturally wise little alien (this is what pictures of babies in the womb most resemble). They seem to have their eyes closed, fervently still attached to the flow of dream/ trance/knowledge that comes through the umbilical cord. Are they trying to make sense somehow of the limitless flood of knowledge that is human history to date? As if it is all flowing in through the cord and they are busy knowing. Knowing everything and plumbing the depths of the mysteries of time. They are concentrating on all of that.*

*Or maybe they are consumed with imagining each little cell and every bit of tissue that will make up their being. This is what I am doing right now. Right now little one ... what should I call you? I have some ideas in mind. The beginning of a shape, a name, maybe even a face ... but I am so afraid to say or even write them. Me, the materialist, the unflinching existentialist. You have terrified me into a state of totemic superstition. That is how badly I want you to stay. Stay with me. Stay with us. Find a cozy spot. Burrow into the blood rich wall of the lining of my womb. Get comfortable in there, make yourself at home.*

*I promise you it will be fun. Why do parents make promises I wonder. How can I promise that? But I do.*

## 32. out of the blue

According to quantum physics everything we perceive as a solid object, even the hardest thing you can imagine, like a rock, is composed of mostly empty space. The only solid things inside each atom are such tiny particles that the amount of solid matter to empty space is about like that of a fly buzzing around in a football stadium. Think about that for a minute. There's your football stadium. Bzzzz ... there's your fly. It's not a lot of solid matter and this begs the question of how or why we human beings perceive things as solid to begin with. Why is it useful to experience this certainty when, in fact, most of the universe is a wash of space and liquid in a permanent state of flux. I am by no means a physicist, but if I had to hazard a guess I would say that it makes us feel better to have an experience of firmament. We are aware of gravity, but we don't perceive surface tension. Our brain simply creates a solid base upon which to stand and this is likely a merciful gift of simplification.

Matter, then, is a useful fiction, and "reality" is whatever an animal needs it to be constructed as in order to survive and thrive. We have trouble imagining the very large, the very small, or the very fast, and this is why our human senses only register a narrow band of available stimuli. In fact at this moment, every possible future exists in possibility. Maybe if I really concentrate I can will this little creature into existence inside me. Picture the single cell dividing and subdividing until — at some point it might be impossible to pin down — sentience begins. Where does that amazing initial spark of life come from? For many years it was supposed that the sperm held the vital substance and that we women were merely a moist fertile swamp in which the elixir was planted to grow and flourish. At one time scientists even imagined that a complete little being existed inside the head of each sperm. I have seen a hilarious line drawing of a fairly mature infant complete with rosy cheeks and cowlick à la 1950s encased in a pollywog shape and swimming furiously toward the goal line. Inside of those creatures they imagined that a multitude of even tinier babies existed, again fully formed. Sperm were seen as nature's version of the nested Russian dolls, each perfectly formed and existing inside its slightly larger version on down to infinity. Maybe matter and reality itself are malleable enough that if I simply will you to be, you will come to be in my belly. I am going to sit here, just sit right now, and try.

## 33. *pluses and minuses*

We have been testing for Viviën's surge for the past few days and the little purple stripe is not appearing according to schedule. We have let our donor know when the window is likely to come. He is an avid hiker and plans rugged climbs and camps, so we are hoping that she won't suddenly start ovulating on a day when he's climbed to the top of the Chief or some other equally precipitous chunk of west coast rock. At this point, if necessary, I am prepared to chase him right to the tippy top of the highest peak, sterile container in hand, and bring back the magic elixir of life. I'll get the special shoes and the rope and the crampons and whatever other pieces of equipment I need and scamper right up there.

The body doesn't always comply with your best made plans. Viviën's surge refuses to come on the appointed day. You can't control this, of course, and stressing about it only makes things worse. So she does an ovulation test each morning, and then we spend a good part of the day working before exploring some new beach or trail with the dog in the late afternoon. The sun beats down, roasting the pine needles until a comforting scent wafts up around us. I've never felt more relaxed and happy about the future.

Meanwhile, I am overdue. I am only one day past my period and I positively feel pregnant. I feel like a huge chemical process is bubbling away in my belly right now. It's as if I can feel cells dividing, but I know your mind can play tricks on you, and I definitely shouldn't count my embryos before they're hatched. Viviën thinks we shouldn't do the test so early this time. It was so emotional last time when we had a positive and then I miscarried very early. I keep picturing the films I have watched of the moment of conception. How, how, how is a person supposed to concentrate at all with one of the universe's grand mysterious chemistry experiments taking place in the cauldron of their belly? Viviën is right, though. We'll wait one more week.

## 34. X's and O's

Today is the day. I peer into the pool of perfectly captured urine in the receptacle in which rests the rocket shaped contours of the pregnancy test stick, whose little plus or minus sign holds the secret of our future. The litmus paper itself is white, and upon it, if we are lucky, will appear a bright purple X. If we did not manage to get pregnant this time, a negative sign will show up in the little window. I try not to watch the stick, try not to count under my breath. I walk out of the bathroom and onto the deck. Viviën is at her computer, working, and I haven't told her that I'm doing the test. I can feel my heart pounding. I can feel the blood making circuits through my body as the seconds tick by. Crickets sing on the wires in the noon heat. An eagle flies back to its nest in the tree top, which, due to the steep banks on the island, is just level with our deck. It has something grasped in its talons. On the otherwise undisturbed expanse of ocean below, a cruise ship, bright blue and white, cuts a line of froth. On our deck, an ant hoisting a huge crumb over its head is making a break for the far side. It crawls over my toe and continues on its urgent journey. I tell myself that when it reaches the other end of the deck I'll go back inside and look at the test. When I stick my head around the door I see it right away. I call Viven and we look at it together: a bright purple X, undeniably dark this time. An X like the X from X's and O's. Her smile warms me all the way to my toes.

## 35. dykes and tykes on bikes

So much for waiting until the three-month mark to let our news out. The icy mountain of our self-restraint melted into a puddle before the blasting hair dryer of our bliss. I am aware of the bellyflop that an unwieldy metaphor makes in a paragraph, but I love it the way mother herons must love their ungainly babies. It's Gay Pride in Vancouver: the best city on earth. Mountains, the sea, beaches, flowers being sold on the sidewalk in front of convenience stores. The West End is bedecked with festive drag queens and lovable leather men. The sea wall is festooned with dancing twinks and dykes sporting ripped t-shirts and asymmetrical haircuts. The air is aflutter with ticker tape and glitter. Free spankings or free hugs (according to preference) are available all up and down Davie and Denman. PFLAG (Parents and Friends of Lesbians and Gays) gets a roar of approval from the crowd as they pass by with their heartwarming signs proclaiming: "Love Makes a Family" and "I love My Gay Son and If You Met Him So Would You!" The Raging Grannies rage no less, though it seems to me their number has dwindled from the red and purple wearing pack I remember from my last Vancouver Pride, years ago. Still, they press on over to Robson in the honey-coloured sunlight of the afternoon. Out on the water, dance tunes pulse and throb as do boatloads of muscled and smoothly depilated sailors. Who doesn't love a man in uniform, right? We munch handfuls of fresh cherries and blueberries while laughter rains down from the rooftops.

All of this combines to make us completely forget our vow to keep to ourselves the news that we're going to have a baby, so we tell the group we are spending Pride with, a mixture of old friends and new ones. They send up a cheer on our behalf that we can hear even over the roar of the tailpipes as the Dykes on Bikes roar by. "Hey, next year you all can be dykes and tykes on bikes!" one of our friends hollers. "Or dykes with tykes on trikes!" yells another.

And it feels so good to tell people after all these months that the dam breaks ... and we tell everyone. We get on the phone to friends overseas, family far and wide ... and then as the day wears on I start spilling the beans to strangers and passersby. "We're going to be mamas!" I call out to two beautiful young men who glide past in blue body paint, hand-in-hand on rollerblades. "That's awesome! Sweet!" They say, and one of them circles around and plants a kiss on my forehead.

## 36. partnering with the floor

Just as a photograph of someone can't really tell you much about the way their face moves in real time, so talking to someone on the telephone can't give you a solid impression of what they are like in the flesh.

Although we've found a donor and I'm already pregnant, we still have a coffee date pending with potential donor from Vancouver Island. He and I had emailed a few times when we were still in Calgary and agreed that we would meet up in the summer. Recently he wrote to me to say that he had a trip planned to the mainland. So we had made the date before all of our recent developments, but also, based on past experiences, we promised ourselves to meet every potential donor who might be a possibility for either one of us.

It is in this spirit that we are meeting in the West End of Vancouver with a dancer from the Island. It happens to be perhaps during the only downpour in a rare hot sunny summer in the Lower Mainland. He texts us and we pick him up at the Skytrain station.

Unfortunately, when I get out of the truck and wave, he spots me and swoops in for the hug right away. Now I'm not by nature a hugger. I don't mean to be a porcupine, and embracing is of course great with long-time friends and family, but I actually loathe the obligatory greeting or farewell embrace. I do it, when needed, out of cultural sensitivity and I will kiss the French on both cheeks. The Dutch require at least three kisses, which raises the question of which cheek to go for first, and I usually miscalculate and knock heads with whomever I am trying to warmly greet. A nosebleed from a clumsy head-butting Canadian is probably not what my Dutch extended family expect, but it's usually the result despite my best intentions.

So when this stranger (who may or may not give us sperm) gives me a hug, it is not a great omen. And his hug is not the preemptory "hi, how's it going" hug either. He cups one huge hand behind my head and nearly lifts me off my feet with a full-body, "I am intent on feeling each of your seven chakras" hug. I have to exercise severe self control to avoid squirming. I see Viviën giving me a sympathetic look through the windshield. I just took one for the team, and we both know it.

The Dancer/Hugger gets in the truck, and small talk commences. We haven't eaten since the night before and I am ravenous for (what else) scrambled eggs, so I ask if he minds if we go to Hamburger Mary's for breakfast. If Hamburger Mary's stop making their Swiss Scramble before I deliver there is a possibility that I will just sit down in the middle of the floor and throw a tantrum. Hamburger Mary's is a bighearted laid-back burger/breakfast joint in the heart of the gay village and I love it. From the gorgeous twinks who arch their backs and flutter their eyelashes in adorable mating dances over the rims of their coffee cups, to the bears who stretch out their legs while dispatching a three-egg omelette and a tall stack, to the older waitresses who call you darlin', to the superdyke server whose entire forearm, back and front, is devoted to a colour portrait of Star Wars C-3P0 in painstaking detail … the whole place just oozes good vibes.

We get settle in and take menus. The Dancer/Hugger doesn't want to eat, which is too bad because I feel awkward trying to chew and talk with someone who refuses to eat something themselves. No matter. In this early stage of pregnancy there are very few food items that are congenial to me, and I am not about to let a little bit of awkwardness get in between me and my eggs.

Viviën is studying the one-page menu for far too long. I decide I need reinforcements and so kick her under the table. She looks up and pitches in. When in doubt, get them to talk about themselves. It is a handy rule you can use in almost any situation and it usually saves the day.

"So, you're a dancer? What kind of dance do you do?" she asks.

"You probably wouldn't know it," The Dancer/Hugger says, waving his hand somewhere above his left ear.

"Oh? What is it, like, salsa dancing or hip hop or tango or modern dance?"

"It's not one of those old style dances. It is called contact improvisation. It doesn't have a style per se."

Not to be put off, she dives in again. "Well what kind of music do you dance to?"

"Actually it's done without music. Most of the time, it's silent." Now The Dancer/Hugger has a kind of long-suffering look as if this isn't the first time he's had to explain his calling to the uninitiated. I sneak delicious bites of soft egg and sip heavenly orange juice. I kind of know where he's going with this.

Before I started writing, I was an actor. I landed quite a few parts with no training whatsoever and started working in Halifax, and then I heard that the National Theatre School was holding local auditions. The school is notoriously hard to get into. They take ten people per year from all across the country, and I was very surprised to get an offer after my first audition. I moved to Montreal and applied myself to the tenets of their training with every ounce of strength in my nineteen-year-old body.

I thought those instructors held the keys to the golden doors of culture and art, and by god I was going to unlock them. I took their teaching as articles of faith, suffering through sessions where our instructors would lock us in a dance studio for movement class. The class consisted of three hours together wearing tights in a chilly room with a wooden floor and mirrors. We were given scanty instructions, such as "breathe in the colour yellow," and then we were supposed to explore movement in response to that. The notion of the minimal instruction was, I suppose, for us to get in touch with our emotions through some kind of "breakthrough." It is to be expected, however, if you lock a bunch of late teens/early twenties theatre students in a room and ask them to find themselves … there is going to be some drama. Capital D Drama. These classes would usually wound up with half of us whooping and loping around in circles, screeching like maddened chimpanzees, and the other half of us on the floor covered in snot in the foetal position and weeping for all we were worth. Occasionally, one person would touch another person. You were meant to take that energy and "move with it." Now that I've had a chance to study a bit of elementary psychology, I not only question the worth of such an endeavour, I find it remarkable that we avoided serious physical violence. This was exactly the kind of murky unspecific ersatz spirituality that put me off actor training.

Looking back I realize that about half of my classmates at some point had a breakdown, which the instructors applauded as a rite of passage for any actor worth their salt. In fact when one of our number had a nervous breakdown, overdosed on sleeping pills and wine coolers, and then slept with a lascivious liver-spotted visiting directing teacher from New York all in the same week, she promptly got the coveted part of Desdemona in our upcoming production.

All this to say that I have experience with the ritualistic talk of some people in the performing arts, so I was less surprised by Dancer/Hugger's responses than Viviën was.

"So do you have a partner that you dance with?" she ventures.

"Actually I don't dance with a partner." He leans forward, places his elbows on the table. I catch a bad whiff of his halitosis and start backward with my elbow protectively sheltering my plate. I worry that my elusive appetite will go south and I won't be able to finish my Swiss Scramble.

"Oh. So no music, and no partner…"

"Well most of the time we partner with the floor."

Viviën's fork actually halts at a dead still at the midway point between her plate and her mouth.

"Sorry, can you say that again? My English is bad. Did you say your partner is the floor?"

"No" he says, a chilly tone colouring his voice, "I said we partner *with* the floor … and sometimes with the wall."

Things slide downhill rapidly. The Dancer/Hugger asks some questions about our life, and soon after hearing about our renovation projects in Holland and Nova Scotia, he wants to know which place we'd like to have "The Father," as he is now comfortably dubbing himself, live in. I am guessing that he hasn't heard the part where we are busily renovating one place and renting out the other, because he's already packing his bags in his head and getting ready to bust out the U-Haul. Alarm bells are going off in my head, and I can practically see Viviën's leg muscles quivering, she wants to jump up and bolt so badly.

"Wait, are you saying you want you to *live* with us?

"I'm eager to cohabitate. I'm happy to relocate, too, for that matter." He leans back in his chair with a sigh and blasts me with more bad breath. He relaxes as if attending his sudden unlooked for but welcome retirement party. Cohabitate? I really don't think so.

When he proposes we spend the rest of the day wandering around Stanley Park in a driving rain storm and getting to know one another better, we backpedal furiously.

"No, we can't. We have things … yes, we have to do this afternoon. Right? Things… " I grasp at straws.

"We're going to look at a condo," Viviën rescues me. And that is true. We're not in any position to buy such a thing but we are going to look at one, so it's a good excuse. But I am now afraid that if he thinks we're buying something on the west coast he'll be even harder to shake off. We ask him where he wants to be dropped off, and he directs us to the public pool in the West End. When we get there, I get out of the truck to say goodbye. Why I can't just stay in the truck and wave good bye? I do not know, but I have some kind of deep devotion to hospitality that was imbedded deep into my psyche in rural Nova Scotia. We might not be moving in with him any time soon, but the man did take time out of his day to come and meet us. He did come into this meeting with ideas and dreams of his own, and I want to say goodbye nicely.

I jump out of the truck and extend my hand. For a shake, I hope against hope. I am not escaping that easily however. Completely ignoring my earnestly outstretched appendage, he comes close and claims his parting full-body hug. Before he releases me, gasping and spluttering from the fumes of dancer-funk that have invaded my nostrils, he loops a woven string with a sachet around my neck.

"This," he says, leaning back, eyes wet with emotion "is sage, the sacred herb of women."

"Thanks," I say, "thanks for the herb." I wiggle away and climb back into the truck, disgruntled as a wet cat. Viviën is smiling through the windshield at me. This is payback for leaving her to chat up the lawyer with the limp handshake, I know it. I leave the flurry of text messages that come in from The Dancer/Hugger over the next few hours unanswered. Apparently he has a completely different idea about how our visit went than we do. And now I wonder sheepishly about what to do with the sage.

Viviën says to chuck it out the window. It's natural so it isn't littering, but I can't quite bring myself to do it. It kicks around on the dash of the car for a few days. Then mysteriously it makes its way inside to the counter, then the kitchen table. Every time I clean up I move the sage and ask myself why I don't just chuck it out. Should we burn it? But is that symbolic of some kind of agreement between us and him? We don't want that. Should we throw it in the sea? But that seems too grand a gesture. Finally we just pour it into the long grass outside the house. When we pass by it smells lovely and we leave it at that.

## 37. letters to possible creatures (kwispelen)

Viviën has started talking to the baby in Dutch. Since she wants a boy, she thinks of "him" in this way already although he is only far enough along to resemble a little fish and hasn't any gender at all. He probably still hasn't lost the tiny tail that embryos have. I joke that when she talks to him, he wags it. In Dutch that action would be *kwispelen*.

"Wait, there, I feel something" I take her hand and move it across my belly. "Yes, there, right there." I swear I can feel a response when she speaks against my belly in her language, the words right against my skin.

For my part, I write another letter to this possible creature.

*Dear Baby To Be,*

*Right now you have a tail. You resemble much more a tiny fish than a human. I read that all of your tiny organs are already there. This seems insane to me, that even a tiny liver, a tiny brain, eyelids and everything should be there in miniature already. This truly seems rabbit out of a hat-like. You have a tail and you are mostly heart. Almost all of you right now is composed of a beating heart. Compared to the rest, the organ is simply huge and the entire body must catch up, grow around and absorb the heart.*

*The fact that we humans start out in life with significantly more heart than brains seems to clarify so many things. We want you very much little one. I try to picture the very first cells of you dividing and subdividing as if I could will you into existence and wonder if this helps.*

## 38. maximum fecundity or Escher stymied

This morning I learned something that made my head spin in a dizzying Möbius strip. You never think of yourself all through your lifetime as having eggs inside of you. Eggs are for sunnyside up, for hatching in the spring or possibly whipping into a nice meringue. Grade A or free range, brown with speckles or creamy white. I never worried about my own eggs in the same way that I did those of the piping plover. (Am I treading on their fragile ecosystem, how will they raise their young between the gangs of stampeding tourists with beer coolers and boogie boards?) In fact I'm pretty sure neither one of us has imagined our own bodies as ecosystems, but now that we're in the process of trying to conceive, suddenly we do. And it is odd. I now imagine my insides and Viviën's as a kind of delicate wetland, a marsh or head waters that could harbour that bright spark of life … or else choke it out in the weeds. I think again of our fertility doctor, who broke it down for us early on.

"Your eggs peak in your early twenties," she'd emitted with quiet assurance. Apparently, after that singular glorious moment of maximum fecundity, your eggs (and every other part of you, no doubt) begin a steady slide. It feels to me now that we've been foolish. If we really wanted to have children we should have started trying to conceive at the age of twenty-three and not a moment later.

"You are born with all the eggs you'll ever have," the doc had said, "and for the rest of your life all they ever do is deteriorate in quality."

At any rate, here is the Möbius strip part: the thing that is even wilder than consideration of yourself as a warehouse for an ever dwindling brooder of eggs. Your baby, if it is a girl child, at eight weeks already has all of the eggs that she will ever have in a lifetime. Wow. Right now I wish M.C. Escher, he of the impossible staircases and the hand that draws the hand, were still with us. I'd love to see him take a crack at this one.

## 39. womb with a view

People have started asking whether we want to "know" or not, meaning do we want the radiologist to reveal the sex of the baby to us. We all take the ability to get a head-to-toe scan of our little ones while they are still on the inside a bit for granted now. In most routine pregnancies you get at least two chances, possibly three depending on your doctor's recommendations, to sneak a peek at your baby before the big day. This has taken the guesswork out of many aspects of the birth process and saved countless lives and prevented a lot of birth complications and suffering for both mother and child.

Here is one of those weird conundrums of scientific research: ultrasound (perhaps one of the most valuable lifesaving technologies of the twentieth century) came right out of military and weapons research for submarines. Without the research "opportunities" provided by World War Two, it is doubtful whether fetal ultrasound technology would have come about so quickly. In another twist in this all too real life-and-death game of snakes and ladders, this same technology now allows unpiloted drones to drop bombs on distant countries while their "pilots" sit in air conditioned flight simulators a half a world away.

It might be a good idea for me to stop reading about pregnancy now, especially since I am battling with bouts of punishing print-induced nausea, but I can't seem to fight the compulsion. In days gone by women of a certain class were kept locked up during pregnancy in order to strictly control what kinds of things they saw or experienced. This was due to a belief called "imprinting." It was thought that if you looked at things of beauty — classically proportioned statues, ionic columns and the like — then this grave and perfect beauty would be stamped indelibly upon the brow of your offspring. A serene walk through a botanical garden or some gazing upon the figure of Adonis would be just the ticket. You were, however, vigorously discouraged from visiting the zoo. Half an hour with the jungle cats is hardly worth junior being born with whiskers, a tail and an appetite for raw meat.

The original beleaguered/celebrated elephant man himself (the inspiration for the famous case study and film) believed until the very end of his life that his appearance was due to imprinting. He had been told that his mother had been startled by a rogue elephant that had escaped from the circus while he was in the womb. Of course now we're much more enlightened. Averting your gaze can't solve everything, right? On the other hand I don't see a need to plan any trips to the zoo anytime soon.

Something else I didn't know before is that babies are often born with fur. I don't mean peach fuzz, I mean a solid coat of fur on their forehead, arms and back. The book I am reading, a term-by-term guide to pregnancy, assures me this is entirely normal. Despite the frequency with which that word crops up, so little of what I've learned about the process seems to apply.

For example, some pregnant women, upon hearing a baby cry, will begin to express milk. Okay that strikes me as flat out weird. A sound-activated milk-o-matic? That's what I'll be in a few months? Phew. Okay breathe, breathe. I am a resourceful and curious dyke of the world. I grew up far outside the strangling bounds of the mainstream and I know strangeness. I have thrived upon oddity, change, flux and uncertainty as amphibians thrive upon the boggy wetlands. What was it the Queen of Hearts scoffed to Alice? *Sometimes I've believed as many as six impossible things before breakfast?* So why not this too?

## 40. ad nauseum

Two words: projectile vomiting. Meisner out.

## 41. letters to possible creatures (dear tadpole)

Today I woke up and smelled the piney earth of the first growth forest baking out in the sunshine after the rain. I looked out over Vancouver as it slowly woke up: this city of steel and glass levitating on the tip of the Pacific Ocean that I fell for so hard in my twenties. Then I flew bedazzled toward the light and I singed the tips of my rural wings. This time I approach from the water. From here on the little island, I can reach across an expanse of water that is familiar to me. Close enough to touch, but with enough salty blue to keep everything in perspective.

*Today I walked outside and I could smell the sentient arbutus that grab the rock and hold the earth together impossibly on the plunging ocean cliffs all around us; I could smell them growing. And I was sure, suddenly, that you would be a boy and that this smell would be the one of your boyish skin after you swim. I imagine this smell coming out of your clothes when I wash them. Emptying your pockets I find beach glass, moth cocoons, mice bones and a live centipede. The spoils of a hard day's work at being six.*

*Yes this earthy scent I can imagine emerging from your clothes when I wash them. Hold on a minute. Wash them. Is this me? Waxing Poetic Over Laundry? Having Dreams of Domesticity? How to reconcile these feelings with those of my younger self who set out hitchhiking (hitchhiking! You could be kidnapped, killed, mangled, worse!) from my little Nova Scotian fishing town. Most girls my age were already hitched, pregnant or on their way to an acceptable career in nursing or retail, but I had all my possessions on my back and a chip on my shoulder about such things — having a little family. Cooking! Pffft! Doing the Laundry! Azzif! Oh how she would have laughed at me. Yet, it hasn't been so long. Fifteen, no, seventeen years. If the young punk I was then with fresh tattoos still warm from the knife and gold spray painted army boots ready to stomp over the whole globe could level a gaze at the woman I've become, she would cock an eyebrow to be sure. See there,* woman. Then I would have smirked at that ungainly term. Rotund it seemed to me then, somehow too fleshy and complacent. The very word woman, itself, in the light that I saw it then, seemed to hold a whiff of giving up and I didn't want to be one. Of course now, after studying women's history, I understand it was the passive stereotype of femininity I wanted to duck, not the powerful term woman. I wonder, tadpole, how will I help you understand all of this. How will I help you grow up strong, and understand that strength has no gender? It doesn't, no matter what they tell you. I will try my best, I promise.

Today I watched helpless, from a hundred metres away, while a three-year-old suddenly burst free of his father's grip and dashed right out into traffic. Tires screeched, hearts were clutched, but there was no impact. The boy looked up, blue eyes laughing and oblivious to what he just avoided as his father snatched him back safely once more. And I felt just a hint of the terror you can only feel for one you love dearer than yourself. That's it. Right there. That will happen on a daily basis, you'll open your calf on a rock, you'll turn both knees to hamburger on the asphalt. You'll climb to heights you shouldn't and tumble down from them too. Oh lord, how will I survive it?

I want to dip you in the river Styx so you will be covered in a barely visible layer of shimmering iridescent bronze through which no ill will, no arrow-head of spit can pierce. But I remember the myths — they echo through the synaptic caverns of memory for each year I have taught them, teased out each nuance of their meaning. They ripple and eddy through my electronic files that accrue for every year I teach the myth of Achilles. If I do this, if I wish for you to be godlike in the Greek or Roman sense, if I think of ways to dip you in this river of (imperviousness) of metallic protection, what does it mean? That even right now, as I write and imagine you whiplashing through a million chemical reactions and little explosions that I already want to start coating you in layer and layers of mother of pearl. I always thought that was a funny expression. The layers of a pearl coat the piece of sand. What does it mean that I want to make you stronger than me? Less vulnerable to pain? From which well could such a desire have sprung. To have a boy, to know a boy, or to be a boy? All of the above?

## 42. bumper sticker logic

The printing on a bumper sticker is like a text tattoo. You might not want these words written on your own vehicle or even less so your own flesh for that matter, but the fact that someone else has committed to them to such a degree tends to give them added weight.

I've only ever found two bumper stickers that I could commit to. The first read "If Mama Ain't Happy, Ain't Nobody Happy" and graced the back of an early eighties Honda that looked like a cross between R2D2 from *Star Wars* and a terra cotta clay pot. To look at it, you'd think it would barely move at all, but that little beast could haul some serious ass. It never quit running on me, and you could drive from Vancouver, B.C., to Lockeport, N.S., on less money than it now takes to buy a decent pair of shoes. That bumper sticker got me chased down by a gay guy in Cape Cod. He was waving his arms so excitedly that at first I thought, damn, I must have cut him off in that long line-up to get off the I-95. I thought he wanted to yell at me, but no. Once I pulled over, he pounded the jamb of his car door in glee, and called, pointing at my bumper: "You have the story, you have the goddamn story of my life on your bumper!" After which he pulled away, still laughing and waving goodbye in the rearview.

My second bumper sticker saved me from a speeding ticket on the far side of Lake Ontario. Although those little towns on the most remote stretch of the Trans-Canada consist of little more than two signs: Welcome to Vermillion and the other saying Thanks for Visiting the Same, you are still meant to slow down to fifty when you pass through them. On one of my east-west road trips I had forgotten to do so when suddenly I saw a police vehicle almost riding my bumper. He flashed his lights. Damn. I pumped the brake and rolled to a stop.

As the Mountie approached I saw that he was smiling. A big toothy grin. Now that is a new one. I fished through the dash for licence and registration and prepared to assume the position. Wait a minute. He was giving me a thumbs up. Now this is definitely a new occurrence. Terrace Bay must be a heck of a place, I thought, even the cops here are nice. Then I realized he's read my bumper sticker, this one gracing my old Toyota hatchback, which read, "Women Want Me, Fish Fear Me." When he drew up level with me, he noticed I'm not a guy. He realized that irony can be deployed on bumper stickers, and I thought oops, I *am* going to get that ticket. It turned out, however, that it was just too awkward for him to sort out, so he let me go with a tight-lipped mutter to "watch my speed." My point is that if something is written on a bumper sticker, people read it, and not only do they read it, they (willingly or unwillingly) give its argument careful consideration. And the bumper sticker that is furrowing my brow today is: *Doulas: Don't give birth without one.*

There's the problem with bumper stickers. They are relentlessly direct. Not — *consider giving birth with one ...* but *don't give birth without one.* What is that — a warning, a threat or merely an admonition? Oh dear. And here I thought it was all about midwives. I have heard of doulas but I have to confess that with everything else going on, I haven't really investigated their role in a birth. The question is, can a bumper sticker hold enough sway over my psyche to make me consider getting one? Yes, it would seem so, because as soon as I get home I run to the closest thing I have to a spiritual advisor: the Oxford English Dictionary online. The handy unassuming interface calmly informs me that the word doula comes from the Ancient Greek δούλη and means "female slave."

O wise Oracle, surely you don't mean that I can't give birth without endorsing a master/servant dialectic? I read on and become steadily more terrified. A doula, it seems, is someone who helps with both the birth process and the death process. That seems like a very wide skill set, and I was kind of hoping to avoid the latter if possible. Okay. I'm eating mountains of vegetables, I've been off alcohol for nearly two years and I've given up sushi. I swapped my high impact sports for brisk walks, and I'm steering clear of stress when possible ... but I think we'll be okay without a doula.

## 43. Wilson

Last night I had a nightmare that the baby came out as a tennis ball. Not just an ordinary tennis ball, but a talking tennis ball reminiscent of Wilson the volleyball, Tom Hanks' only companion on a desert island in the movie *Cast Away*. In the dream I am trying to get the tennis ball to clamp onto my breast to nurse. I am using the proper angle and murmuring encouragement but it is very frustrating. The baby refuses to feed and bounces off down the hallway and out the door with a reckless grin. When I wake up, I am utterly distraught because I think the baby is a tennis ball — a disobedient tennis ball, no less, and completely heedless of his own personal safety. Until my head clears, I am in a heart-racing and soupy stomached state of panic. As bedside reading I have been attacking *From Here to Maternity,* a book given to us by our doctor. It is five hundred pages and is only one of a tall stack sitting by the bed. I do want to do my due diligence and follow best practices on this whole birth thing ... but I think I'll have to swap the reading material up for something else just before bed.

## 44. trying again in Peachland with a separated rib

If at all possible we still want to keep trying for Viviën to conceive a baby with the help of our current donor. Now that we are back in Calgary and he is still in Vancouver, this operation has become tricky. Whereas before we only had to navigate the relatively calm stretch of Howe Sound in order to get the magic elixir, now we have to get over the Rocky Mountains within a day of detecting her ovulation surge. The differing lengths of her cycle make it impossible to book a flight in advance.

Our donor, going far above and beyond the call of duty, agrees to drive to meet us halfway, in Kamloops or some other Rocky Mountain town. If there were an award for acts of valour and kindness toward infertile couples, he would be a shoo-in at this point. But then we get a message from him saying that he's been rear-ended in a car accident. Although he's avoided major injuries he does have a rib separated from his sternum. This sounds quite painful and means he can't drive. It is Wednesday and Viviën should ovulate any day now. Although the situation has become more difficult, we let our donor know that we are not giving up. We'll come to him. We'll drive all the way over the Rockies if need be.

We are in standby mode. All we have to do is get the little purple line on the pee stick and we are all set to jump in the car. In the midst of the confusion, Viviën keeps forgetting to test her urine.

"Oops!" she says, clapping a hand to her forehead after emerging from the bathroom, having forgotten to collect a urine sample, and so I keep plying her with glasses of water.

"What am I going to have to do here, stake out the bathrooms? Seal all the toilets with duct tape?"

Just as we are starting to lose the light on Sunday afternoon, I hear a whoop from the bathroom. She's got a stripe. We call our donor and he says he can take a bus and meet us half way between Vancouver and Calgary. He has friends that live in Peachland, and he will take the bus out to visit them for a night. We pile ourselves and the dog into the car and head west into the setting sun. The drive over the mountains is a bit wearying, considering all of the travel we have done in the last little while. As Viviën settles herself in behind the wheel, it occurs to me, not for the first time, just how many adjustments she's made to be here with me.

It's not just the tyranny of hearing only English spoken, the inhospitable climate, uniform architecture and lack of decent cheese. Viviën also had to become accustomed to the very different Canadian sense of space and distance. You can drive the length and breadth of Holland in a couple hours, yet most Dutch never do. The cultural differences between Rotterdam and Utrecht are huge, but you can hop from one to the other in less than an hour unless you hit the dreaded traffic jam or "file." Then there's no telling how long you'll be stuck. Canadians, on the other hand, will drive twelve hours to get away for a long weekend. We'll do Calgary to Edmonton to have lunch with a friend. To give something the designation "road trip" you need to pack survival equipment and plan to be gone for a couple weeks. It requires a portion of your life.

One of the first times Viviën came to visit me, we hopped in my little pick-up truck and drove from Nova Scotia to Alberta. For one reason or another, I seem to do this east-west mega trip every year or so, but she must have found it utterly surreal. Crossing the Maritimes alone is the equivalent of driving across Holland, Belgium and France … and you haven't even hit the maddening and never-ending single-lane highway around the top of the great lakes.

By now Viviën is somewhat used to long road trips, so setting out in the late afternoon to drive to the next province, particularly for such an important errand, doesn't seem to strike her as all that strange. The sun blasts in our eyes for the first few hours. It is the end of summer, with the first hint of yellow fire at the tips of leaves that announces autumn. It is hot and sticky, and as we soon discover, it is peach season in Peachland. If you ever find yourself in the position of having to drive to Peachland for sperm, I recommend that you go at peach harvest time. The whole place glows in lambent shades of peach. The wasps are maddened by the scent of fruit that is so ripe it nearly splits its own skin. We stop and get a barrel of peaches and they are succulent. The juices run down our arms when we bite into them and the fuzz is exquisite. As we drive, we see pickers stalking up and down the aisles of the orchards, baskets slung over one arm. The crisp, sugary aroma hangs even in the night air as we drive along the highway — a long sinew of blue/green lake on one side and orchards on the other. We can't eat all the fruit we buy and decide that when we get home we'll make jam. Then this winter when we are frost bitten and buried in snow we can open a jar and have a little taste of Peachland in August.

When we finally arrive it is after eleven. I am once again astounded and grateful for the good will of our donor. He answers his phone on the second ring and says that he'll be waiting for us outside the hotel in five minutes. It is hard to put my gratitude at this moment into words. It is a very strange feeling, to say the least, to have an almost stranger do you this favour. A gift that could, no ... that already has, changed the course of our lives. And how do you repay someone for this? Maybe the answer is quite simply that you cannot. Ever. Like the beauty of the little boy's questions that I admired some time ago, the gift exists not to incur a debt. It exists for its own sake and has a logic and a beauty all its own.

Having been through the process already with him, things are a bit more comfortable this time. I leave Vivën and our donor to chat in the car while I check into our hotel. We drop our things inside quickly since it is late. After a very quick chat, Vivën and I take the dog for a walk to give our donor some privacy. We barely make it halfway around the block when Rockit lifts his ears and then takes off after a skunk that he spies across the cracked asphalt of the empty hotel parking lot. I call him back frantically. A tragically stinky dog and a trip to the Seven-Eleven to buy them out of tomato juice could add an unwanted chapter to this evening's proceedings.

*Do you want to bath the dog in tomato juice or give the sperm donor a lift home?* I picture us asking one another in a not-so-classic debate. We are great at division of labour, even when it borders on the absurd. A text message comes in on Viviën's phone that reads *All done,* and the dog breaks off his chase just in the nick of time. When we arrive back at the hotel, our donor offers to give us another donation in the morning so that we can try again and double our chances. I am very grateful to him and very impressed with how at ease he is in his own body and how forthrightly he treats this great favour he is doing us.

I marvel at all of us, actually, for this modern and reasonable arrangement. We have not let geography, biology or really anything stand in the way of the family we want to create. If something is truly important to you ... you can't afford to let anything stop you.

Now all we have to do is wait and find out if this attempt is successful and if Viviën is carrying our second child. We hadn't really thought about this scenario. After hearing the odds from the fertility specialist we assumed that we would be lucky if one of us was able to conceive a baby. *But what if we get double pregnant?* I picture us both waddling along hand-in-hand with two big beautiful bellies taking the lead. Who will tie the shoelaces? Who will pick up anything that gets dropped? What about when we check into the hospital? What will it be like to help one another give birth?

*Breathe, breathe! Now, push, honey, push.*

*I am breathing, you push, yourself, dammit!*

One crucial difference will be, I guess, that we'll never be able to say to one another (as I've often heard women say to their husbands): You have no idea how this feels.


## 45. lucky

Although I've been a student and a teacher of women's history for some time, I am quite surprised about how little I have gleaned to date about how women actually manage to bring new humans into the world, both in the present day and throughout history. Trying to correct this glaring oversight, I gather information wildly, from documentary to anecdotal. Any information is valuable as long as it is about the process of giving birth.

Some women fairly glow when they talk about giving birth. Not just the part afterward where you get an amazing little baby to love forever, either. The actual process. They frown upon the way that giving birth has been over-medicalized. They tell me not to anticipate pain but rather to think of it only as intensity. These are the women who plan to or have already given birth in kiddie pools in their living room with no further pain relief than an advanced pregnancy yoga position and deep breathing. They are calm, self-assured and serene. These women frighten me.

Then there are the women like Viviën's very forthright Polish sister-in-law, who, when we asked her how she found the process of giving birth, reported: "Imagine squeezing a watermelon through your nostril, and you'll have some idea what it feels like to give birth," which was also quite horrifying in a different way.

No matter where you stand on best practices for birthing (home birth or hospital, midwife or doctor), there is no question that having a baby at this point in time in Canada makes you one of the lucky ones.

At certain moments of history, and still in some parts of the world, giving birth is a kind of calculated risk. The dice being rolled with the lives of mother and child. This is often compounded by the fear/distrust with which patriarchal systems treat women's bodies. The rhetoric of chastity has made it difficult for doctors to study women's bodies with anything like neutrality. Contemporaries of Ignaz Semmelweis (1818–1865) thought he was peddling subversive and superstitious hogwash when he suggested that doctors wash their hands before attending women in childbirth, and yet this simple act dramatically reduced the number of women dying from childbed fever.

Even the ancient Greeks, whom I love for their refreshingly forthright notions about the body and sexuality and their comparatively strong female characters, had their fair share of lunacy when faced with female anatomy. In the gynaecological treatises of the *Hippocratic Corpus*, Plato helpfully outlines the perils of the "wandering womb" syndrome. This was handily employed to explain any complaint a woman might have. The assumption was that since women were both the source of life and the root of all evil, then the female reproductive organs must be evil squared. Got a back ache? Your womb must have floated back there and is causing the problem. Got a bung knee? Certainly that pesky womb must have dropped down there and is kicking up a fuss. Are you stark raving crackers mad? It is likely that your uterus has migrated up to your head and is squeezing off the blood supply to the brain. Oh those dangerous, lurking, troublesome wandering wombs.

Despite the centuries of experimentation upon women and the obsessive study of women's reproductive organs, it was a long time before anyone actually thought of studying semen. Soon after Antonie van Leeuwenhoek invented the microscope in 1676, he got the idea to examine his own semen and discovered millions of vigorously swimming spermatozoa. He was careful, in his report to the Royal Society, to note how he had examined only what, without sinfully defiling himself, remained as residue after conjugal coitus. Sure, Antonie, you stick to that story. Who can blame him? Scientists, especially when they are really onto something big, have to cover their asses. Look what they did to Galileo. Luckily the Royal Society saw fit to accept van Leeuwenhoek's explanation, but the part that sperm plays in reproduction took another hundred years to be verified. Lazzaro Spallanzani, an Italian priest/scientist, managed the minor miracle of getting both permission and financial support from the Catholic Church to study sperm. Most of his work was with frogs, so perhaps this helped. He observed how the male frogs fertilized the strings of female eggs in order to make tadpoles. He made tiny oilskin prophylactic trousers for the male frogs and put them on during the mating (that must have been a trick in itself), after which no tadpoles occurred.

Now that we could be pregnant to the power of two, the household interest in all things reproductive has increased exponentially. In fact, it is pretty difficult to focus on anything else in this crucial period before we can do a home pregnancy test for Viviën and while we ride out the waiting period before I can have an ultrasound. We sit down together to watch an acclaimed BBC documentary on the history of childbirth, which has the effect of making us feel very fortunate to be able to give birth at the beginning of the twenty-first century in a democratic country in the "developed" world. This documentary points out the horrible irony that the very doctors who were sworn to protect women in the past were often the ones to endanger them most.

Modern western medicine may not be perfect, but I am reasonably confident that I will be able to enter the hospital and give birth without anyone fumigating my genitals with scorched insects (a treatment popular in the Medieval Period), nor practising bloodletting, nor locking me in a room for a few days before checking to see how it all turned out.

## 46. Pachelbel or Hendrix?

Even though the tiny creature in my belly doesn't yet have ears but only tiny flaps of skin or maybe proto-ears … and the perhaps (and much hoped for) being in Viviën's belly hasn't even those yet … I am playing a lot of classical music. Experts recommend that classical music be played for babies in the womb. Studies show that their growing neurons can be fed with the repetitive arrangements in classical music. While the jury is still out about whether a steady diet of Mozart will actually result in a measurable increase in creativity, mathematical skills or spatial awareness, the experts are fairly sure that listening to classical music never did anyone any harm.

Those experts probably didn't sit through the gory beige-pancake-makeup overstuffed version of *Salome* on the world's most uncomfortable opera stool in a sweaty little cubicle with the grumpy Austrian critic that I did this past summer, but no matter. Experts are experts, and at this uncertain stage of pregnancy, I find the dulcet tones of certainty reassuring. I flip through our CD collection looking for something responsibly baroque yet not too sombre. No need to depress the wee mites at this early stage. Pachelbel's Canon in D major. I suppose it would be cheating to use Coolio's remix, so I stick with the original. I've read that everything you experience, in some mysterious chemical way, is passed on to the embryo in your tummy, and so I am looking for ways to stay on an even keel. I tried yoga but I want to throw up as soon as my eyes leave the horizon, so that is a tough one. Yesterday, on the phone from Nova Scotia, my mother told me that she had been reading about a woman who put headphones on her tummy while the baby was still in the womb.

"Oh yeah," I said. "What happened, did the child emerge a musical prodigy? Was she calling for sheet music and a metronome before she could chew solid food?"

"No, but after the baby was born she was very fussy and nothing would put her to sleep. What the woman discovered is that if she put on some classical music the baby went right to sleep. Worked like a charm."

My mother is my go-to source on these matters. She is reassuringly practical and one heck of a good parent herself. I quite like this application of high culture as soporific so I resolve to give it a try. I take out some old-school five-pound headphones and clamp them onto my now slightly protuberant belly. It looks frankly hilarious. And I don't want to risk damaging emerging eardrums so I take them off and just play the music out loud.

After about fifteen minutes, I am sucked back into another century — in a less than pleasant way. I can feel the drafts coming around the castle walls causing the tapestries to flap. Behind the lapping waves of fervour I hear the counterpoint of chains of lost souls of the damned clanking in the basement. Vivïen calls from her office upstairs asking if I can please turn down "that noise."

I stop the CD and quickly replace it with the next one in my very idiosyncratic filing system. *The Collected Works of Jimi Hendrix.* Immediately my ears say thank you. Unfortunately, researchers haven't yet done the much-needed study on the beneficial effects of Jimi's sophisticated feedback harmonics on the developing mind of the unborn child. I lie back on the sofa resolving to write a letter to some editor somewhere urging correction of this glaring oversight. At the correct volume, with speakers that allow for texture and complexity, Hendrix holds up to any piece of classical music I've heard. And as a bonus, there are the lyrics. I listen to Jimi assure us: *You can hear happiness staggering on down the street, footprints dressed in red, and the wind whispers Mary.*

I wonder what he means. I wonder if, in fifteen years or so, I'll be able to put this same song on whatever kind of system we'll use for music in the future and ponder this same question with our children. Will we ask each other what Jimi meant? There is symbolism in the red feet, surely, but why is happiness staggering? Maybe it is in the nature of happiness to stagger. Will we all scratch our heads together over that one? I hope so. Or maybe they'll say: *Oh Ma, you're so weird.* That'd be okay too, I think. I can hear Vivïen working at her desk upstairs as I drop off into a blissful nap.

## 47. training for it

I have noticed that people are much more familiar with you once they find out you are pregnant. What was formerly a part of your body now becomes public property. The overly exuberant will rub your belly while the more restrained will limit themselves to reaming you with information about the birth process complete with graphic accounts of hideous pain or blissed out epiphanies, depending on the source. There is a real move right now toward home birth and some women will almost wrestle you to the floor and put you in a head lock if you tell them you are thinking of going to the hospital. I've been treated to a few diatribes condemning modern science for pathologizing what should be a natural experience.

I do understand that the historical mistrust and fear of the power of fertility has often played itself out painfully upon the bodies and spirits of women and that the medical system (just like the legal and political systems) is reluctant to give women full enfranchisement. I get that. One male friend even told me that he believed that doctors and health care professionals have created a culture of pain around the birth experience. He was of the opinion that the word pain should never be used in conjunction with childbirth. We should always use the word intensity. He assured me that most women, with the right guidance and care, are able to achieve orgasm during the birth process.

Choosing a metaphor that appeals to my athletic side, he went on to compare giving birth to a marathon. You wouldn't go out and try to run a marathon without training for it he said with an air of finality and at the time it sounded quite compelling. Now that I think about it, what exactly can I do that would qualify as training? *You* put five pounds of baby and another ten pounds of fluid under the skin of *your* abdomen then go out for a nice twenty-four-kilometre jog while trying to keep down your bland breakfast against a vicious onslaught of morning sickness, I want to tell him. I have trained up to marathon distance and run the half in a fairly decent time and I just don't think the analogy works. While running itself and even running for long distances is indeed within the realm of natural human activity, there is nothing about completing a marathon that is natural. Even high level professional athletes who are trained to a perfect pitch still know that completing the race equals damage to their bodies. The body is not designed to run a marathon. Once you pass the eighteen mile mark you have burned up all the fuel that your body is able to store. You can try to replenish with sports drinks or gels but the body is not built to digest at the same time you are on the move. What happens when you run out of fuel, but you keep on running is that you begin to burn up your own fat, protein and even your own muscle tissue. The body begins to use itself for fuel.

Scientists have now found that most marathon runners, even elite ones, suffer tiny tears and ruptures to their heart during the race. There are micro-fractures to the bones. These wounds might heal. You might consider them worth it, in the face of the sense of accomplishment you get at the finish line. That is all fine. Athletes test their bodies all the time. The whole point is to push yourself over the limit. But to do that while you have another life inside you is just plain nuts. Every fibre of my being says no to extremity right now. I want moderation. Bland food. Walks up the side of the cliff with the dog in the open, fresh air. Frequent naps. It sounds boring, but this is exactly what my body needs. Anything else and it rebels. I am put right down forcibly on the sofa by nausea.

It's not a good idea to cultivate dread. Dread causes stress and stress sends all kinds of bad chemicals coursing through the blood stream. But this emancipatory theorizing about natural birth needs to be balanced out with the fact that women first had to storm the pharmacy doors for access to medication for pain relief during childbirth. Giving pain relief during childbirth, of course, for most of history has been avoided as it was thought that women brought forth children in pain as a kind of penance. If there's one thing that reading a lot of history will do for you, it is to lessen the point of your absolute certainty and create a mental climate of useful self-doubt.

## 48. control is a thing you learn to lose

This morning Viviën comes down the stairs with a huge smile on her face and hiding something behind her back. It can only be one thing and I run over to see. Yes! There it is! Our second little gorgeous purple x in the window of the pregnancy test. This is really happening. We are double pregnant and our little family is set to, very suddenly, double in size.

For the next week or so we toss around baby names. A name is a tricky thing. It can't be too ordinary. I know from my attendance sheets at school the chagrin of all those Johns and Cathys as they share their name with a third of the class. On the other hand, a name like River or and Rain kind of screams *It's not my fault my folks are hippies*. Finally, we have the added challenge that the names have to sound good in both English and Dutch. And this turns out to more complicated than you might think.

"What about Leo for a boy?" I ask and Viviën shakes her head.

"It sounds very old-fashioned in Dutch."

We rule out names that echo natural phenomena and names with silent, half-pronounced or unpronounced letters. A child saddled with Eionan or Charion might spend hours — maybe even weeks or months over the course of their life — correcting other people's mispronunciations and misspellings. Time they will never get back.

Despite my critical view of the way gender functions in mainstream society, I don't think it is a good idea to name a boy Sue, as in a song my grandmother used to play on her eight track. Maybe he would be building character as he climbs out of the school dumpster the angry mob stuffed him in, but I don't think he'd see it that way at the time. Viviën points out astutely that this type of cruelty can always happen and it doesn't depend on a name. Kids try out behaviours like mean and dumb just as they try out everything else. The terrifying and icy thought presents itself … no matter how hard you try, you can't ever fully protect them.

Excellent point. In light of that perhaps it is better to confront them with the facts of life early. Maybe we should go with a boy named Sue. Or perhaps naming him after a cheese would do the trick. Viviën likes the dignified British ring of Stilton while I am leaning toward the fiery Italian cheeses.

"What's your name?"

"Pecorino Romano," he'll sigh wearily, rolling up his sleeves for the sixth time in a week. "We can just do a scuffle now, or I can pencil you in for a full-on fist fight after school."

You probably can't choose the magic name which will guarantee that your kid won't get picked on at school. Another part of the big lesson: control is a thing that you have to learn to lose on a daily basis. As the inimitable Elizabeth Bishop put it in one of my favourite poems of all time: *The art of losing isn't hard to master; so many things seem filled with the intent to be lost that their loss is no disaster.*

## 49. fear itself

This is, I suppose, the pinch of non-fiction. Right now is when, as a playwright, I would love to snuggle deep into the blanket of anonymity that writing with a cast of characters gives me. The "I" feels too naked and helpless to stand up to the hot lava scorching through my guts. Fear. *There is nothing to fear except fear itself.* This is not helpful, FDR or Francis Bacon, whichever of you truly coined this syllogism. Because fear itself is scary. The news we just got is so devastating that I can barely take it in. I don't know if I have the guts to keep writing if things go badly.

We go in for our first ultrasound. A kind young student squirts cold gel over my belly and zooms the ultrasound wand all over. When she presses down, a fuzzy image appears out of pixellated points of light and there he is. Or she. Tiny perfect hands and feet. Lying with one arm draped across his forehead — for all the world same way I sleep. The sleeping posture Viviën teases me about, saying that my elbow pokes her in the ear all night. The baby is there — alive, reclining, healthy — and turns over as if being awoken by the ultrasound from a pleasant nap.

I know that the baby's movements at this point are all involuntary; they function to develop the muscles and nerves… But it seems like the little one is saying, "alright, enough already" at a certain point. Viviën holds my hand between two of hers as if it were a delicate, breakable object. We are astounded at this, our first look at the little creature that our love, determination, and the kindness of a stranger has created. The student performing the ultrasound gives way to an experienced technician, who pokes and prods far less gingerly in order to get the pictures and measurements she needs. The baby, she says, is large for his age and everything looks good. We are to wait outside to get formal results from a nurse.

We sit there amazed and grinning at each other for about fifteen minutes until the nurse calls us in. I notice immediately that something is off in her manner. Her shoulders are cinched up, and her face has a determined and professional cant to it that sends a shiver through me. "The baby appears fine on the ultrasound."

*Appears*, the way she says the word catches on me like a piece of barbed wire. What does that mean, appears? Suddenly I am an animal with its foot in a steel trap. I want to rip the word apart, shred it with my teeth and hands. The nurse looks at her chart and not at me. She can't look at me while she says that levels of certain substances in my blood are out of whack. The PAP is low and the HGH is high. If the acronyms are familiar to you, then perhaps you already have a chill running up your spine. If they aren't familiar, then you'll be feeling the same bafflement that I did puzzling over these things for the first time. The upshot of all the screening and testing is that while many types of chromosomal abnormalities have screened negative, it seems there is a one in twenty-two chance that our baby has Down Syndrome, Trisome 18 or another life threatening genetic defect. This number is elementally terrifying. The picture that leaps into my mind is a classroom. My classroom. Twenty-two isn't even a large class.

The nurse tries to put it in perspective for us. She knows that news of this sort is difficult to hear. It is, however, basically an algorithm completed by a bloodless machine that combines my maternal age with the imbalances in my blood and has dealt us a hand grenade for a statistic. I can hear her voice. Everything she says is going right into my brain almost as text, and I see her mouth moving but the room has pitched sideways. I hear a hungry howling wind inside my head.

She outlines the options for us. Two types of invasive tests, both of which carry a risk to the baby. The first of these is a CVS, or chorionic villus sampling, a frankly terrifyingly procedure where a doctor passes a needle through your belly or a tube through your vagina and cervix in order to snip out a tiny piece of the chorionic villi: these are the little finger-like projections on the placenta. The cells there can be analyzed to tell practically everything about the baby from the sex to the chromosomal make-up. The pain and tension of the test aside, the procedure itself carries a chance of spontaneous miscarriage.

To add another layer of difficulty to the decision about whether to go through with a test such as this, I am already in my thirteenth week. The nurse encourages us to consider what we would do with the information, if we get it. Would we choose to end the pregnancy if the results of the tests uncover a serious problem? If we do want to end the pregnancy we have to decide quickly as the date is rapidly approaching beyond which an abortion cannot be performed. We would need to start making bookings this week. It is difficult, she says, as the waiting list is long to book me for a CVS. We need to decide now if we want to get on the list. If we take even one day to think about it, then the waiting list itself would probably take us past the window of decision-making about whether to carry the baby to term.

To be faced with this kind of choice, on the spot, is overwhelming. I am trying to keep the logical part of my brain working as I know our family's future depends on it, but I am rapidly melting down. We ask for a moment alone and talk about what to do. When the nurse steps out, we decide to book the test, and then go home and talk about it. We can always cancel if that is our decision, but if we don't book it, the decision could be taken out of our hands.

Intense quiet envelopes the truck as we drive away. I have to walk into class and teach in an hour. Not just a ninety-minute class either, a three hour evening class, the first one of the term. I would like to cancel, but to do so would effectively rob the students of an entire week of instruction. Also it is in the first class that students gather most of their impressions about the value of the course to them and unconsciously calculate how much effort they will put into it. So even though I feel like a wreck of a human being, I lock myself in my office, force down some juice and bread, and get ready to walk in there.

I have planned an introduction to ancient Greek comedy — material close to my heart, and yet I can feel my usual enthusiasm for the roots of comedy failing me. The first comedies were essentially an extension of fertility celebrations — complete with cavorting actors dressed as satyrs wearing outsize phalli and bushy tails. I usually love to teach this stuff. Students are often shocked to find out that today's society is composed of blushing violets when compared with the classical Athenians. For the first time in my life I feel leaden and funereal while elaborating points that usually bring down the house.

Fifty pounds of worrisome concrete sit on each shoulder as the class limps along. Despite this, I can still see sparking glints of interest. These almost ephemeral moments are a lifeline to any teacher. It is this ineffable quality of live teaching that makes teaching possible at all. One of the students begins holding forth on the subversive power of humour in the hands of the underdog. We linger over the damaging effects of the laughter of superiority when it is practised by a dominant group upon a scapegoat. An example is given, a comparison made, as we dig into connections between the satyr play and modern satire. We talk about the physical benefits of laughter, how endorphins released by humour can aid in healing and produce benefits to health and well-being. The students are smiling and laughing as they filter out into the hallway. Almost without effort from me, it seems, the class is launched.

## 50. crossing the bridge

My response to the news is to bury myself in research. I have a deep and abiding trust in the power of knowledge. I grew up in a struggling little Maritime town as the fisheries collapsed, and my mother raised me alone. She worked four or five part-time jobs all through my youth to make ends meet. She grew up in a family of fourteen children who lost their father, the captain of a fishing boat, to the sea. Although the family was filled with clever and promising individuals, they all had to go directly into the workforce. It was a challenge to finish high school, and university was out of the question.

It was the one article of faith at our house that school was my way out. I had to get out, and in order to get out, I had to go to university. In order to afford university, I had to get scholarships. In order to get scholarships, I had to bury myself in books for most of my young life. I did all of the above, and in spite of all the valid criticisms that folks have about the Ivory Tower aspect of education, books are the security blanket I run back to when needed.

When threatened, some creatures thrust their heads inside their hard protective shells. Some gulp air and swell to eight times their natural size with spines protruding and face the attacker. Still others slap the water with their tail as a warning and then swim to safety. I read. And read and read and read. I begin to learn about the way the medical system uses statistics and numbers upon people in our situation. In the process I devour every book available on pregnancy and gain an understanding of the silent suffering women have to endure in the present and in nearly every historical era. Until finally, I feel it with a stab. *Knowing doesn't help.* What a ragged, threadbare blanket knowledge is in a real storm. Knowledge doesn't keep you warm or safe; in fact the more I read, the more I break out in chills and cold sweat.

Finally Viviën grabs me and the statistics and turns us both around. The chances are still ninety-six percent that the baby is totally healthy, she says. And furthermore, she knows that he is. How? She just knows, she *feels* it. "Ask yourself," she says, not letting go of my shoulders, "do you feel like there's anything wrong with our baby?" And I take a moment … and ask the question. Ask it directly to the little creature inside me: *Are you okay?* And somehow silently, I get the answer.

He's fine. We are not doing any of those tests. This simple act — it never would have occurred to me to do it, as I have a kind of brain lock when it comes to numbers. Numbers are like the point of a knife sometimes, the way they can efface the humanity and emotion of a situation and convert it to digits. How can we introduce risk into his still fledgling life for the sole purpose of giving ourselves a hundred percent peace of mind. What a ludicrous fantasy of humanity's ability to reign supreme over nature. A delusion of mastery that isn't worth the danger it introduces.

There is no foolproof plan, no guarantee of safety. Now it begins to make sense to me that in some cultures, when a woman becomes pregnant, a celebration is prepared for the dawning of a new life, but they also prepare for a potential death. This double helix can't be unwound with DNA analysis, blood tests or 4D ultrasounds. We want to see and to know everything. We want to haul all of the mystery out into the open and make it safe … but it's impossible.

We talk to a genetic counsellor, who is wonderfully calm and tells us that this is only a screening based on statistics, not a test. She says that having a CVS with my numbers would be venturing into the territory of alarmist. We talk about several options, and she recommends a "marker" ultrasound at week eighteen. They look specifically for developmental signs of Down Syndrome, things such as the lack of a nasal bone or irregularities in the bowel. If we have that test, and nothing turns up, then she says our risk is cut in half again. It has the benefit of zero risk for the baby and for me: no needles, no chance of miscarriage or deformity. It is also, she says, not too close to the wire. I ask what the wire is, and she elaborates that if any "markers" were to turn up, we would still have time to do amniocentesis. This is another needle, but about half as risky as a CVS, and it would show definitively if any chromosomal problems are present. They would get us in very quickly for this test, she assures me, perhaps even the same day. This would still leave time, under the law in the province of Alberta, to terminate the pregnancy, if that is what we choose to do. Even with the absolutely professional and neutral tone she is using, even with her careful sanitization of the language, I can't choke down the lump of inky panic in my throat.

I am terrified but promise Viviën that I won't worry, because I know that sometimes stress and worry can do more harm to the baby than the thing you're worrying about. How's that for paradox? Also she is at a very delicate stage of pregnancy herself, and what if this stress and worry impacts the baby she is carrying as well? But the mind is a creature that isn't easily tamed by simple promises. When I lie down at night thoughts come back like vicious little hyenas worrying at my heels. Viviën is sleeping and she needs her rest. She is making our little daughter or son. I will myself to lie still, not to twist and turn and disturb her. I need to read. Bathe in narrative. Lose myself in another writer's words, until words swim across the page and blend with my first dream. It's the only way I've ever learned to get to sleep. Turning on a light, even my tiniest covert book light, is to risk waking her up. I must be able to go to sleep some other way.

No, the hyenas snap, snarl and chew. I beat myself up for worrying … then worry that beating myself up for worrying is really only another type of worrying, worrying to the power of ten, probably, and that this stress too, can be communicated to the fetus through the placenta.

*I'm sorry. I'm sorry, little ones. I'm sorry Viviën. I'm just a sorry sack tonight who can't stand the contemplation that the darkness brings.* I ease my bulky body over to the edge of the bed. I angle the reading lamp so that it gives off just enough light for me to make out the page. I open the Naomi Wolf book *Misconceptions*, which a colleague kindly gave me when I passed on the news that I was pregnant. Wolf quotes an African proverb that says giving birth is like going across a bridge. Your loved ones can send you off with warmth, can wish you well and can be waiting for you on the other side, but the crossing … the crossing you have to do alone.

## 51. smallmedium@large

We have begun to let people know that we're starting a family, collecting hearty congratulations and best wishes on all sides. We decide to make the trip to Edmonton to visit my best friend, confidante and critic. I could use the term "ex" but it doesn't begin to cover what we have meant to one another and still do. Ex gives the idea that someone very important could be suddenly erased or crossed out of your life. This just doesn't happen. Love doesn't go away, but it can change shape on you. Just because you have ended one dimension of the relationship (physical intimacy, cohabitation), so much else can still remain.

We have, treading carefully, erected a sturdy friendship over the remains of a seven-year love relationship. For first time, she has invited some members of her family to share the visit, her brother and niece, who I was very close to. It is so great to see them again. Her niece has now passed from a precocious kid with an ear for the absurd to a lovely young woman in her first year of university, and the spark of originality and sensitivity that I remember remains. The smile of my friend's brother, who has recently been through several life changes of his own, tells me he is at ease and ready to reconnect.

During the course of the dinner party, one of my friend's new acquaintances reveals her occupation and also her particular skill. She is a small wiry woman with that patented two-tone spiky-dyke haircut — short and unruly, with several longer pieces and a shock of blonde on the forelock. Her day job, she tells us, is to do the clean-up at messy crime scenes. *Yikes.* I think. Her gift and skill set, however, are quite different; she reveals to us without a blink that she is psychic.

It takes a moment to digest the implications of what seem to be two occupations entirely at odds with one another. It must mean that while she cleans up the blood and the guts and the physical spillage of lives that have been destroyed, she can also feel (and has to cope with) the psychic spillage of those unfortunate endings. *Double yikes*, I think, biting the inside of my cheek. I have the urge to giggle but not because it is funny. I have never been a new-age person, nor particularly atavistic. On the other hand, I do have enough of my Maritime grandmother in me that I have a healthy respect for superstition. I won't knowingly walk under ladders or let a black cat cross my path. I don't willingly step on cracks in sidewalks, and I go out of my way not to break mirrors. I figure, if there is any such thing as karma or fate or what have you, there's no point in getting on its bad side.

Additionally, this compact woman has flashing eyes and a lot of presence. She is compelling. In response to a flurry of questions from the room, she is remarkably down to earth. She must be quizzed all the time about this, but she is patient. She acknowledges that it is difficult, in her situation, dealing with the psychic fallout of the crime scene. My friend suggests that she could be wasting her talents in this environment. Maybe she should set herself up in business independently and solve the crimes before they even occur. Heck, why stop at crime prevention, she could branch out to any number of fields. She could have a website called smallmedium@large. I laugh, as do the small woman herself and the others at the party.

And yet, when we are leaving for the evening, the small medium allows everyone else to filter out first, until just she and I are left in the room. This near-stranger bends down and kisses my protruding belly through the thick wool of my fisherman knit sweater. This, for me, would usually be deeply weird. Given the chance, I might even pull back, but she is fast. She reaches down and cups my developing baby paunch before I can retreat. She looks into my eyes and says: "Both you and the baby are going to be fine. There's no reason for you to worry about that."

This is very odd because no one at the party, in fact no one at all outside of Viviën and me, knows anything about the test results and the worry they've been causing us. Now certainly these could be generic words that the small medium says to all pregnant women. But, how can I say this ... they aren't. And for once, instead of making a joke that tucks

129

everything into a folder for my intellectual self to classify later, I feel tears well up in my eyes and I let them. "Thank you," I say, "thank you so much," and I throw my arms around her.

## 52. sublime bean

I am attending the Under Western Skies conference here in Calgary. This cross-disciplinary meeting is bringing together activists, academics, artists and people from the non-profit and government sectors to focus on the environment. At the moment a sprightly academic with requisite tweed elbow patches is spending his allotted twenty minutes trying to wrestle the notion of the sublime to the ground with his bare hands. It is, he says, being in the presence of beauty that simultaneously strikes awe into your heart and scares the crap out of you. That could be an irresponsible paraphrase on my part, but I seem to be experiencing what I've heard other pregnant women jokingly call "placenta brain." This condition causes you to forget handy facts and historical dates that usually come to mind with no problem. It causes you to forget where you parked your car, what it was you wanted to buy at the supermarket and, in extreme cases, your own birthday.

What, from a certain perspective could be seen as absentmindedness, from another, perhaps Darwinian, point of view, could be regarded as a useful narrowing of focus. Parts of your brain that normally deal with any number of high-level functions are temporarily colonized and are now only concerned with the impending arrival of your baby. It's a very useful adaptation, this, to ensure the survival and continued well-being of this precious and helpless tiny creature.

Placenta brain aside, I still attempt to follow the lecture. The sublime, Elbow Pads insists in a breathy voice, is "well-meaning ineptitude that rises to empyreal absurdity." I write it down here on my notepad because I have absolutely no idea what that phrase means. This doesn't usually happen to me. I am accustomed, by employing a bit of concentration, to being able to wring at least the bare-bone meaning out of any English phrase. It gives me a weird feeling of freefall when I look down at my pad and register almost nothing. *"Well meaning ineptitude that rises to empyreal absurdity"* I read again. Nothing. Come on brain, ignition! I can almost smell burning rubber from the effort but still nothing.

"I want a scone," insists placenta brain, in survival mode, and against my will my gaze wanders from the speaker over to the snack table. I plan my attack. I can make my way over there between speakers, I decide, charting a course between the chairs full of conference attendees that will admit my increased girth. I used to be light on my feet, athletic, I could have woven through the sea of listening faces even during the lecture without raising a stir. I could have retrieved my desired scone and a cup of coffee and returned to my spot, all without disturbing a soul and all the while conveying to the speaker on the podium that I was still absolutely engaged and listening. If I try to make my way over there right now, it will be like a seal lolloping through a beach full of sleeping birds. It is difficult not being able to fit in any of the places you used to fit into.

"Sublime," says the speaker, "is being in the presence of the quality of greatness or vast magnitude."

"I still want that scone," throws in placenta brain, but I focus on what the speaker is saying. This is precisely how I felt this morning when the young radiologist squirted cold jelly all over Viviën's just-beginning to-show beautiful round belly. As the ultrasound wand glided across her and squiggly lines of black and white static swam on the overhead screen, I put my hand on Viviën's leg. The radiologist in training was having trouble finding the proper signal. The lines assembled and dissolved frustratingly as if capturing that mysterious moment where a bunch of cells in the primordial soup of the womb are suddenly infused with electricity and start to pulse in unison.

*Oh, there!* I said as I spotted the tiny intricate creature in Viviën's belly. We looked up at the monitor for our first look at our second baby. Just the size of a bean and slightly curled in upon itself. The baby was cradled along the bottom of Viviën's womb, and we could see the little heart hammering in bright bursts three times per second. I could feel my own heart beat faster in response. The fact that we've already seen one of our babies via ultrasound did nothing to diminish the sheer sense of mystery and wonder.

"Sublime," says the speaker again, "going back to basics, from the Latin *sublimis* (looking up from under) toward something high, lofty, elevated or exalted." And suddenly I get it. You're right, Mr. Elbow Pads. I feel a hundred feet tall. As tiny as a grain of sand. Brave. Strong. Protective. Terrified. There in the tiny radiology room with my hand on Viviën's warm thigh and her smile bursting out suddenly when the little bean appeared, I was in the presence of the sublime.

## 53. why do they call it morning sickness

Viviën is so sick. Just knocked out for most of the day and hardly able to eat. Sure the nausea starts in the morning, but to call it morning sickness is really to imply relief at some point in the afternoon, which is simply wishful thinking. The thing about having gone through these stages two months before she does is that I know what she's in for. I offer some things she might be able to keep down. Yogurt? Ginger ale? She is used to being strong and able. Being knocked out in the middle of the day for no good reason is at first a horrible feeling when you can usually put in a good eight or ten hours of physical work. But I found that trying to fight it only made it worse. I tell her this as I head out to work in the morning. "You are doing one of the most important pieces of construction work in your life right now. It's just that you can't see any of it. It's all happening inside your belly."

She smiles at this and looks pale.

## 54. boy business

Ultrasound number two for me brings us a very lengthy session with a student radiologist who, despite copious amounts of cold jelly and an hour of belly poking, cannot seem to get any clear pictures. To be fair, the baby isn't making it easy for her. Every time she clicks the button an arm or a leg flies up and covers the face. I know that the way budding radiologists become full-fledged ones is precisely this kind of practice. I don't mind submitting to a little extra poking and cold jelly for the common good. The only problem is that we've been waiting in a kind of desperate forced calm for these results. This more detailed, or "marker," ultrasound should give us an indication if anything is wrong.

The student happily pokes away, getting, from what I can see, about two million shots of the baby's kidney but not much else. I am pretty anxious to talk to somebody about the results of this ultrasound, and I ask, "Will someone come to talk to us about the results right away, or do we go to the waiting room first?"

"Uh … don't know. Sit tight one minute, I can't get a good picture. I have to talk to the radiologist and the doctor." And she leaves.

Vivïën holds my hand and we gaze at the magical creature up there on the screen. Hands and feet moving ever so slightly with the fluid ease of a sea anemone. Two feet crossed at the ankles and one hand draped over the face as if playing peek-a-boo. We don't say much, we are just waiting for an all-clear. We've remained calm for the last few weeks. We've been taking vitamins, we've eaten vegetables religiously, and we've been even more than exceptionally kind to one another. What we want is for someone in a white coat to tell us that everything's going to be okay.

Another radiologist comes in. She is slightly older, with tattoos and dramatic eye makeup, like a goth kid who grew up and found a profession. Without saying a word she shifts me over slightly and gives my belly a good solid poke, and the baby, as if on cue, turns over and stretches out to be photographed.

"There we go. They're afraid to do that, when they first start," she says, "but there's no way you could hurt them with a little poke," and her face opens into a smile. Snap, snap, snap. Like a prenatal paparazzi, she has everything she needs in a minute flat. Suddenly she turns away from me and zeros in on Vivïën.

"You look scared," she says to Vivïën, which sounds odd as the words strike the air.

"No, I'm not scared," Vivïën says, "we've just been here for a while."

"We had some blood levels that were out of whack. This ultrasound should tell us if everything is okay," I add.

"Well you have to talk to the doctor, of course. But everything looked good to me. Good luck you two. You can get dressed and go to the waiting room. They'll call you in for the results," she says heading for the door.

"Can you tell if we have a boy or a girl?" I ask.

"Oh yeah, that's easy to check. Sure you want to know beforehand?"

"Yes!" Viviën and I say in unison.

"The trainee didn't tell you?"

"No!"

The grown-up goth radiologist zooms the wand over my belly again for what seems like a split second. Her eyes are much more practised than mine. All I can see is sonar snow.

"Aha! Of course we never make definitive predictions at this stage," she says, "but that looks like boy business there, to me." And then with a flip of her jet-black and fire-red bangs, she is gone.

Boy business! We're having a boy, we tell each other in the odd glow of the ultrasound room. I am so happy. We are going to have a son. A little boy. Viviën will hoist him up on her shoulders and ruffle his hair and teach him to weld and do a crossover dribble. Of course she could also teach all those things to a girl. In fact she still might. Who knows what the future holds?

We still have to go into a conference room and discuss the results. We won't be out of the permanent state of emergency until a doctor takes off the hex that was put on three weeks ago. They call my name and point us toward a tiny room with one comfortable chair. Viviën and I each try to nudge the other toward the chair with the cushioning. We wait for what feels like three years. Outside the door I hear the doctor joking around with someone. He is telling a story that sounds like it is going to take a while before it reaches the pay off. Of course it isn't right to feel impatient. He has the right to enjoy his day and to exchange pleasantries with his coworkers. But we have been waiting for three weeks for these crucial findings that could impact the entire life of our baby. Finally the story winds up with a smattering of laughter and the door opens.

"Which one of you is Ms. Meisner?" asks the thin doctor with a thick Irish brogue. I put up my hand as if I'm in class.

"That would be me. But I'm a Mrs."

"Are you now," says the doctor and looks at Viviën pointedly. "Friends, then?" he asks her in a hostile tone. He puts such an accusatory spin on the word that it seems to wobble and lose its meaning. *I'm guessing you have precious few of those*, I want to tell him. Or *Sure, Doc. Really good friends, with benefits.* There are a hundred ways to resist the doctor's homophobic bedside manner but right now we can't focus on anything except the piece of paper he is holding in his hand. The one with our little one's future written on it.

"We're married," I say calmly, but I can feel a little creak in my voice, "to each other." He stares down at our important results paper and acts as if I haven't said anything at all. At this a storm cloud crosses Viviën's beautiful features. If this was any guy on the street being disrespectful about our union, she would send him scurrying away, tail between his legs ... but this man is sitting on information we need.

"Well, the baby's measuring up beautifully. Everything seems normal." He still does not let us see the paper, and he rakes his eyes over us scornfully as if to say: *Yes, everything seems normal ... except you two knocked-up lesbians from outer space.* We make a few more inquiries about the markers that this ultrasound was supposed to check for. The baby's nasal bone is present and well formed. The bowels and heart and lungs and kidney and every other delicate little internal organ too seem to be just fine. I start to breathe. Pins and needles prickle as the blood flows back into my hands and feet. I realize I have been holding my breath for nearly three weeks. Viviën reaches over and takes my hand, and we walk out swinging our hands together in sheer relief.

## 55. oxytocin cocktail

Most mornings now, one of us wakes the other up on one of many trips to the bathroom. That's something I wasn't ready for. Just how many times per day a pregnant woman has to pee. With everything else going on in there I am guessing that my bladder is currently the size of a thimble. Yet with this dry prairie air and forced air heating, I need to drink water all day. I wouldn't like to tally up how much time I've lost in the bathroom. It is after 9 a.m. I am sleeping these days like it was an Olympic sport. I debate between a soak in the tub or a couple of hours' work in my pajamas before heading to the office. This is one of the fringe benefits of being a professor. You might be working like a dog come marking time, but that you can do a goodly portion of your work in your PJs makes up for a lot. If I am going straight to the university, I usually spring out of bed, pound back the coffee and barge right into the day.

Viviën calls me back to bed. Being a lazy Leo she prefers to wake up slowly, stretch and ease into the day. She tells me about a dream she just had. It was a kind of a sexy dream, apparently, in which I made her go and cover all the windows to ensure we had privacy before we could make love. Well, that beats the hell out of the bath. That beats the hell out of working on the computer in your pajamas! I slip back into the bed. The frame is steel that she welded herself, and the headboard is made from a clear-stained piece of purpleheart wood.

Here is something no one tells you about. The utter strangeness of making love and having another little creature there inside you. There is no such thing as alone any more. Perhaps there never will be again. At least not for a very long time. In *What to Expect When You're Expecting* they tell you your baby will taste what you taste, though milder, through the amniotic fluid. They tell you your baby will share the benefits of gentle exercise, their heart rate and blood circulation speeding up along with your own. They don't tell you, however, that when you make love your baby could turn a full somersault inside your belly. No, they don't mention that, and they neatly duck the problem of describing just how strange that will feel. Of course a baby won't have any "memory" of events, but he will certainly get the benefits of all the good natural hormones. He gets to greet the morning with an oxytocin cocktail and a somersault.

## 56. call the networks

There is a distinct possibility that I have been overindulging in television detective shows. Other than playoff basketball or well-made documentaries, I don't usually watch much television. Yet the kind of tiredness that has hit me in the first trimester sometimes makes it challenging to do anything else. I think it goes beyond mere distraction, however. There is something very appealing, on a structural level, about these shows from the point of view of someone who feels their physical capabilities to be compromised. A bad guy is introduced who menaces an innocent victim. Yikes! But then the good guys pursue, capture and, if you're lucky, smack around the bad guy before putting him in jail. When I turn on the television, this pattern repeats itself no matter what channel or what network. It happens every time like clockwork, and if you feel, as I do, that your increasing girth might inhibit your natural ability to flee from predators, this pattern is quite soothing. That is, if you close your eyes while uniformly pretty girls in perfect white lab coats tweeze skin and hair out of gruesome places under the harsh blue light of the forensics lab.

So perhaps I have been watching a few too many of these shows because this morning I dreamed that we, Vivïen and I, were ... get ready for it ... a pregnant lesbian crime-fighting duo. Yes, we were a crackerjack gun-toting, bomb-defusing team of two, ripping through some unnamed yet glamorous international cities in a Ferrari (hey, it's my dream) taking names and kicking ass. Until we finally cornered a nefarious bad guy in his flat. He was in there, we knew it. All we had to do was to kick down the door, search all the rooms, covering each other with very snazzy guns, and then cuff him. Suddenly I remembered that we both have bellies sticking out a foot and a half.

"Wait, babe!" I said to Vivïen, who had her gun at her shoulder and was backing off a few paces getting ready to kick the door in.

"You can't go kicking in doors. You're pregnant." Then I ran up the street, found a very sturdy looking young man and convinced him to come over and help us out. "Would you kindly kick that door in for us? You'd be doing your community a great service by collaring the kingpin of an international drug ring. And you'd also be doing a favour for two pregnant ladies. That's good karma squared." The kind Italian man (I had been, all this time, speaking flawless Italian, so I gather we're in Rome) ran his hands through his lustrous blue/black hair, considered ... and then obliged. He flattened the door with one solid blow of his shoulder. We thanked him, apprehended the kingpin, then went for Vietnamese spicy noodle soup, which she'd been craving.

When I wake up this morning, I tell the dream to Vivïen, who suggests that I call the networks and try to get it into development. Hey CBC, I have a sure-fire new hit for you: Pregnant Lesbian Crime Fighters. What do you think? I'll get to work right away on the pilot.

## 57. letters to possible creatures (on how you came to be)

You were conceived in love with the twinkling lights of the city reflected in the harbour. You were thought of and dreamed about over great distances. Mythic mountains moved so that you could come to be. Over the inky magical water of the Georgia Strait. From the topmost corner, room 802, of the storied Sylvia Hotel.

Whenever I used to dream of being a terrifying literary lioness who kept the world at bay from a slightly aging yet dignified ocean-side hotel, it was at the Sylvia. Yet now my life is taking a different turn. Why did I ever think that you had to lock yourself away from the world to write? Despite the successes of the women's movement, there were still comparatively few women authors on the syllabi of my courses in university. The women writers that we did study appeared to live solitary lives with a monastic devotion to their art. It seemed proof positive that diapers and literature don't mix. As I studied history, I began to understand how women's invisible labour in nurturing and facilitating everything impacted their lives.

You go try to keep everyone's socks darned and tip a literary paradigm on its ear at the same time. I saw how women are often interrupted. How they are hardly ever left to ponder the imponderables, to venture into the belly of the beast and emerge with a glimmering fragment of a crucial new idea. I thought, as a woman, you had to keep yourself safe from the poison of family life. And somehow this image of myself began to set. I pictured myself as a fierce, fiery-eyed writer who kept herself free of the clinging vine. I would avoid the trappings of materialism and the distractions of running a house by living in a hotel. In the Sylvia I would peacefully lead a life devoted to books and literature.

How could I have ever thought that to write you have to lock yourself away from all that is organic? You can't. Now, I know that you can't, and any attempt to sequester yourself from the world is both fruitless and misguided. This is the very stuff of feeling and of books. The very stuff of life itself.

## 58. the belly says no

Although Viviën has been quite strong and cheerful through her pregnancy, today she is in the grip of nausea and headaches. She knows she must eat, but as it goes with nausea, there is nothing appealing enough to get it down. The only really safe thing are those dry Wasa wheat crackers with a tiny smear of butter and a ghostly thin slice of cheese. This morning, seeing that wan, queasy look that I recognize well, I don't ask her what she wants for breakfast. I just make some of these and put them on her desk near her elbow.

Yesterday we had steak for dinner, usually her favourite. Suddenly she looked at it and started to gag. It was noodle soup, only noodle soup, that she could imagine eating, ever imagine eating again in her life. We dropped everything and ran out the door to our favourite Vietnamese restaurant. I know, unfortunately, exactly how she is feeling. Whatever the belly says yes to, you have to gobble it down quickly, before the belly changes its mind.

## 59. the old wives say

Your protective instincts for the life inside you can wreak havoc on your peace of mind. In the last couple of days, Viviën has been worrying that she can't feel the baby moving. I tell her that the ultrasound was fine. We could see the beautiful little baby developing, moving and even turning over. I tell her, squaring my shoulders, that I am absolutely certain our baby is fine. She gives me a weak smile but says she can't feel any movement. Nothing reassures her.

I feel an acid fear in the back of my throat but know it is my job to stay calm right now. It is important to be conscious of the way that the pregnancy hormones can elevate your emotions. Our doctor even told us to try and keep in mind how we might impact each another with these mutual waves of emotions.

I rack my brain for a way to comfort her and finally resort to the old wives method. There are likely worse folks to consult in a situation such as this. I tell her to lie down on the bed, string a needle on a long thread, then carefully let the tip of the needle touch the skin of her showing belly. As you pull the needle up you must be careful to hold your hand steady so as not to influence its movement. The old wives say that if you are going to have a girl, it swings in a circle, and if you are going to have a boy, it swings back and forth.

I'm not sure how it works, but it does. Maybe there is a magnetic force emanating from the little life inside you that the needle picks up. As the needle starts to move, it is hard to tell exactly if it is swinging back and forth or around in a circle, but what we care about most is that it is moving. It is swinging mightily and with no encouragement from me. It is so amazing: our little baby in there. I lie down beside Viviën, place a kiss on her belly and begin to whisper to the baby about all the fun we're going to have together.

*Every morning when we wake up I will look at you and I will say: Today is the start of another fun day. I will, I promise.*

## 60. the sweetest drumbeat in the world

Today we go to see our birth doctor for the first time. Our family doctor told us that she thinks we'll really like the birth doctor she's recommending and that she is "a character." Our family doctor is a sweet young thing originally from Nova Scotia. Being familiar with the polite indirectness of Nova Scotians, I wonder if "character" is code for lesbian, and I kind of hope so. At this stage, there are very few personages that would make me feel safer than a big butch doctor with a buzz cut, an air of authority and a cool stethoscope.

When we arrive, I have a brief flicker of disappointment. Her shoes give it away: little black leather slip-on ballet type shoes with a low heel and bows on the toes. No lesbian would wear such shoes, but as soon as our birth doctor starts to speak, my initial disappointment fades. Shoes and gender identity notwithstanding, she is perfect: energetic, smart, comfortable with us as a couple and sharp as a tack. She finds our case an engaging change from the routine. We tell her how we managed our conceptions ourselves using a known donor, and her face lights up.

Somehow she makes being the object of study an utterly comfortable experience. She does our case histories one after the other and doesn't mind that we want to do the appointments together. We learn that we have exactly the same blood pressure and blood type. Despite the handy fact that we could give one another a transfusion in a pinch (hoping to avoid this sort of a pinch, naturally), we are pleased about this internal commonality, made even more poignant by the fact that on the outside we look completely different.

The doc asks Viviën if she wants to hop up on the table so we can try and listen for the baby. Viviën is a bit hesitant because she is only at twelve weeks and this is a borderline time. Sometimes you hear the heartbeat at this stage and sometimes you don't. Two days ago our GP tried to find the heartbeat and couldn't. Although she showered reassurances upon us that this is normal, normal, normal ... it still brought our hearts to our throats.

I can see that Viviën isn't sure she wants to try because she doesn't want to hear silence again. But I have already checked out the ultrasound equipment in our birth doctor's office. It appears to be newer and more specialized, and so I give Viviën a little nudge and point to it. I really want to hear that steady little hammer, the sound of a life under construction.

Viviën nods and then stretches out on the table. She has her eyes closed as the doc says this will be a little cold and squirts a worm of jelly on her belly. As the doctor moves the wand around, we can't hear anything, and I can see the lines at the edge of Viviën's eyes and lips turn down in worry. "Here," says the doc, "we have to roll these jeans down further and really get in there. At this stage, what they like to do is to hide way down ... here!" Boom, boom, boom, boom, boom, boom! Suddenly the room is filled with the sweetest drumbeat in the world. "A hundred and fifty-two beats per minute, that's lovely, just perfect," says the doc with the tone of a woman absolutely in love with her chosen profession, her kind intelligent eyes dancing behind quirky cat-eye classes. Yes, she'll do. She absolutely is a character, and she'll help us through this next part just fine.

## 61. measuring up like a twenty-year-old

After the scare we went through last time, Viviën and I are braced for the worst when we go for her first-trimester ultrasound. She is a couple of years older than me, and from what we have gathered, everyone over thirty-five is automatically given an elevated risk factor for chromosomal abnormalities. We are steeled for what could be another harrowing round of decision-making about invasive testing.

This morning Viviën told me about a really bizarre dream she had. She had given birth to a little girl, except she wasn't a baby per se. She was a very small, perfectly proportioned person who looked, dressed and spoke like an adult. In the dream, the "baby" and I sat at the dinner table talking about poetry and politics, and we both seemed to find this normal, but Viviën was shocked into silence. Suddenly she looked at Viviën and said, "Why are you so quiet?"

When Viviën asked her if she was hungry, she said yes but seemed to expect a regular adult dinner: "Filet mignon, mesclun salad and a glass of Perrier would be great." We explained to her that she was a newborn and that all the health professionals recommended that she be breastfed for six months. She tried it, but then spat the milk out, saying, "Okay, I guess I'm not as hungry as I thought, thanks."

At first I burst out laughing at the absurdity of the dream, until I see that, even though she knows it was funny, it is also really bothering Viviën. I tell her not to worry, it's normal to have strange dreams in pregnancy. The word, however, feels weird as it comes out of my mouth. Almost every bizarre and disturbing thing that happens to you during this process is routinely categorized as "normal." And the word itself has disturbing implications. "Normal" has historically been used as a kind of disciplining measuring stick — either that or the baton of the police state.

But I am a good wife, and I think something like this is what she needs to hear in order to get through the day. "You're not putting this in the book," she insists, and I quickly change the subject because I know I won't be able to resist doing just that. We drive across the frozen Calgary landscape. The year's first cold snap has come on a full month before actual winter begins and the choke cherries are frozen right on the trees. They would tinkle and break like glass if you touched them. Through the car window I see sparrows peppering the afternoon sky. I can't imagine how they stay airborne. Why don't they freeze and plummet to earth like tiny ninja throwing stars?

We make our way at a snail's pace through stoplight after stoplight across the city. Trails of vapour rise from houses and office buildings, and ice crystals hang to fairytale length from rooftops. We arrive at the radiology clinic and try to make it from the car to the foyer before our eyelashes freeze together.

Within five minutes, we are looking at our baby on the ultrasound, lying peacefully in a soft bed of placenta as if it were a cozy goose-down comforter. As we watch, a tiny fist quivers in front of the baby's face. We can see tiny feet doing leg presses against the inside of Viviën's uterus. By now we know what the numbers mean as they flash up in the screen, and I put my hand along Viviën's arm. The most crucial measurement is the nuchal fold. This is a bit of liquid on the back of the baby's neck, and its measurement gives all kinds of clues as to how the baby will develop. The normal range (there's the fearful word again) is from about 1.5 mm to 2.5 mm, so when I see the numbers up at 1.9 and 2, I breathe a sigh of relief.

The radiologist tells us she is done and that we can head out for a brief chat with the nurse, but everything looks great. The nurse who meets us afterward is apple-cheeked and happy to deliver the news that everything is better than great. "You're measuring up like a twenty-year-old!" she tells Viviën, giving her a good-natured slap on the back.

Now, to a woman at our stage of life this statement is wonderful to hear, even if it is referring to some mystical and invisible chemical balance in your blood. A smile breaks over Viviën's face, and she has an incredible smile, so powerful that when you are standing in the force of it, it feels as if you have your face toward the sun, which has suddenly appeared from behind a cloud. The nurse smiles too and is unreservedly and genuinely happy for us. It must be gratifying to be the bearer of good news, and she beams at us when we tell her that we are a couple and that I am pregnant as well.

It is a funny thing, this moment when we explain our situation to a stranger. Perhaps because we are talking about something as raw as the creation of life, perhaps because it takes people by surprise … there is a kind of frozen moment when their social mask slips off and I can see in a flicker what they really think. In some cases it is wonderful. A person you might think of as conservative or curmudgeonly suddenly opens right up with warmth and surprises you. On the other hand, it can be a let-down. That casual acquaintance or person at work whom you could have sworn wished you well reveals a flash of distaste or worse. I don't mean to, I don't look for it, but it is there as plain to me as a stop sign or a scrawl of graffiti that I can't help but read.

We walk out of the clinic to the car. "Measuring up like a twenty-year-old," I say to Viviën, wanting to hear it again out loud, and the bubble of her relief is palpable, warming us during the freezing the walk to the car and lasting all the way back home.

## 62. gayby boom

According to newspaper and magazine articles, more and more gay people are having children than ever before. Not just those who come out of straight marriages with children from former partners, but also those with a same-sex partner who start from scratch. We are, the headlines proclaim, in the middle of an epidemic; they are calling it the "gayby boom." This could be true. Quite a few of the lesbians we've met out here near the Rockies have kids. For example, we know two hockey-crazed boys whose mums watch their games from the bleachers sipping hot chocolate and organizing stuff via their cell phones during time-outs. Viviën and I are really hoping to join the sports-mums ranks but would prefer it if our kids play sports that take place above freezing and at times that fall within normal waking hours. I suppose if we somehow conceive and raise a hockey fanatic despite our own clear preference for basketball, we'll be in there elbowing and drinking hot chocolate with the rest of the hockey mums, gay and straight.

When I tell one of my good friends (another ex to whom the term does not apply), a painter originally from France but now living in Capo Verde, about our double pregnancy she is ecstatic for us and immediately tells me that she and her partner also want to try and have a baby with a donor. In fact, they have already been trying for some time to find one. It is strange that, even though we keep in touch regularly and talk about our work, we somehow both neglected to share this rather large bit of news until now.

She has a string of questions for me, and I remember this feeling since I had them myself. There are the various medical considerations, such as blood type compatibility and a couple of rogue viruses that aren't so harmful to big people but are pretty tricky for fetuses. Then there are all of the legal and ethical issues that relate to the donor. How much does he expect or want to be involved? Do you want to open your door to him at any time or do you want to organize regular times for visits? Their situation is even more complicated because being gay in Capo Verde, as I understand it, is no picnic. Whenever I get completely fed up with the unforgiving minus-thirty climate of the Canadian prairie, I remember the pain in my friend's voice when she tells me that she and her long-time girlfriend can't live together, can't hold hands in public. They can't even admit to being a couple, not even to their families or their closest friends, who would disown them if they knew. They could lose their jobs, or worse. The stakes really are that high, and there is no system of rights to back them up should anyone discriminate against them or hurt them for being together.

My friend says that she and her girlfriend did have a conversation with one fellow that they worked up the courage to ask if he would consider being their donor. He thought about it, but in the end decided that his conscience would not allow him to create a child who would grow up in a gay household. And this fellow would be singled out from his peers for his progressive attitude just for the fact that he had considered their proposition and drank a tea with them to discuss it. I can't imagine how they deal with this judgement on a daily basis. I can't imagine how it must have felt for them to lose their only prospect for a donor. Because it has proven next to impossible for them to find a donor where they are living, their next plan is for my friend to fly to Paris and meet up with a stranger they have been emailing who has agreed to give them sperm. Of course, this isn't as easy as it sounds. Each attempt involves a break from her work and the timing of an international flight to coincide with her ovulation window, and finally, they are at the mercy of the donor's schedule. They can't afford to both leave Capo Verde this time and so my friend is soliciting advice before she gathers her resolve to go alone to an anonymous Parisian hotel room and make herself pregnant with a vial of sperm from a stranger. My friend is a lovely and intelligent woman, a very talented painter, and I know she has so much to offer a child.

When I hear her story, I feel keenly aware of all the options we have here. There might be a gayby boom, but it only stretches over the parts of the earth that have legal rights and protections for gay people, and that is still a relatively small piece of the globe.

"Don't you give up, you," I tell her on the phone. "You are a brave, brave woman." And I cross my fingers for my friend, her lover and the little child they might have together. Such a child might be the best hope for the future, surrounded by love and poised between the comfort in his own skin and kin and the culture that refuses to accept them.

## 63. jaws of life

It is getting quite difficult to fit into all of the places where I used to fit. Trying to slide between the row of desks and the lecture podium I become momentarily wedged, and the students, smiling, tip their desks back to free me. Getting up from any soft surface is often the culmination of two or three tries. Hold in your mind's eye for a moment the picture of a walrus doing an ab crunch and you're in the ballpark. I have switched over entirely to pants with stretchy front panels, while Viviën, though she now sports a definite belly, is staving off maternity clothes for as long as possible. It isn't the stretchy panels that she minds but the saccharine style; the matronly cuts and fake mother-of-pearl buttons are definitely not her. With each passing week, she just wears her regular jeans a centimetre or so lower so that her belly can grow out over the top. When we are in the kitchen together making dinner now it is a rather tight fit. I joke that if we open the dishwasher or the refrigerator, that is it. We are stuck until the fire department arrives with the jaws of life.

## 64. stay put till we get back to the ocean

After a serious breakfast of reckoning we outline a plan for the next year. We have weighed all the options in terms of where we want to have the babies and spend the first few months of their lives. We briefly consider going to Holland, but since we both have medical insurance here and only Viviën does over there, we rule it out. My work only pays for a leave of twelve weeks, but I simply can't imagine going back to work full-time and leaving Viviën to handle both babies after three months. Also, I don't want to miss this important time in their young lives. Federal maternity leave allows a parent one full year off, but the benefits work out to under half of my regular salary. We decide that if we go back to Nova Scotia and live in our little summer house we'll be able to manage financially for the year.

This means living for a whole year in the small town I so desperately wanted to escape as a young person. My nightmare as a teenager was to be living in a saltbox house in a fishing port, barefoot and pregnant. Now I am making enthusiastic plans to head east and do just that. It is dizzy-making if you start to think about how your dreams and desires can spin you full circle.

Our plan is to live in our now-renovated house on the ocean. I will care for both babies and write my opus while Viviën embarks on another renovation project up the street. At regular intervals she'll take breaks to breastfeed of course. The only thing standing in the way of this admittedly optimistic plan is 3000 miles of wintery Trans-Canada highway and our pregnant bellies. We have a GPS and a map with X's marking every single hospital along the route. The trip will happen within weeks of my actual due date, and this gives me pause. What if the baby decides to arrive early and I have to birth him in the passenger seat in Northern Ontario and cut the umbilical cord with my own teeth? Okay, breathe. Breathe. Best not to contemplate extreme scenarios. Instead I have a serious talk with the little boy nested in my belly. Just sit tight until we get to Nova Scotia, I tell him. We are fisherfolk, son, stay put until we get back to the ocean.

## 65. cosmic weights and balances

Viviën has been certain all through her pregnancy that the baby she is carrying is a girl. Today, when the radiologist swings the wand between our baby's legs I catch a glimpse of what looks to me like boy business. I don't want to interrupt the important work of determining that the baby's little heart and lungs are pumping at the proper speed, but after she is done, I ask if she can see the sex of the baby. She takes a moment to investigate and tells us that, while she never gives out guarantees, it looks to her like we have another baby boy on the way. Viviën seems shocked and doesn't say a word. The pink Adidas hightops she picked up yesterday will have to find another home. On the other hand, why not start his countercultural training early? "Yes, I am wearing pink Adidas," I picture him saying to the other babies. "I trust that no one, in this day and age, is going to have a problem with that?"

In the evening we have some friends over. They are a lovely couple who, though they live like we do, in the prairies, would fit right in on Vancouver Island. They volunteer at the animal shelter in their spare time and they socialize feral cats in their own home. They have a giant iron and glass goddess statue on their front lawn, which is no doubt the talking piece of their block in small-town Alberta, and are also training themselves in various healing and Shamanic practices.

We decide to tell them that we are going to have two sons. It is always great to share that kind of news in person, instead of over the phone with family and friends in another time zone. Viviën is still getting used to the idea of us having another boy. Our friends have brought us some lovely mum-to-be gifts: tangerines, baklava and organic bath salts. They also tell us about an idea they learned recently in one of their workshops. The idea is that perhaps the babies chose us. I am paraphrasing them, but the core of it is that all these little personalities or souls or beings are floating around in a big cloud in the ether. They look down and choose which parents they want to spend this particular lifetime with. In fact, each of us went through this process before we were born and will continue to repeat it, again and again. Neither Viviën nor I spend time thinking about the afterlife or reincarnation, but as a pregnant woman, I have to admit that this notion has a certain appeal.

While at first I thought it would be nice to have both a daughter and a son, I know such preferences probably mean nothing the moment you see your own real live baby. I think I can be a good mother of sons, and I know Viviën will be outstanding. I love to get out there and throw a ball around and have always been a bit of a ruffian at heart. Also, my own life has been marked over the last few years with the losses of boys and men. One of my dear uncles died recently and far too early, and my younger cousin, whom I wrote of earlier, died at twenty-two. My own father has been a distant figure in my life so far and my maternal grandfather was lost at sea before I was born. Maybe, extending our friends' logic a bit further, more boys are just what we need, and the arrival of these two young males in our lives will serve to restore some set of cosmic weights and balances that we can't fully comprehend.

## 66. should old acquaintance be forgot

We made grand plans to celebrate this New Year properly by dressing up these protuberant bellies, taking them out for a nice dinner, and then dancing until midnight. Far from dancing the night away, however, I am holding it down from a comfy perch in the oversized recliner at a friend's house party. I do have a noise-maker at my side, and I am determined not to doze off before ringing in this year that marks the biggest change in my life to date.

Besides, this is no ordinary house party. This is the annual New Year's celebration hosted by a couple of Calgary's original lesbian super mums. They live on an acreage and have a large circle of lesbian friends who also have children. Every New Year's Eve they have a bonfire and a kids-versus-mums pond-hockey grudge match. This is becoming more and more perilous for the mums as the years go by. We lesbians tend to be serious about our sports, and the rivalry has been intensifying as the kids reach beyond peewee and into bantam. Although hockey isn't my sport of choice, I can stop a puck so I usually play nets for the mums. Ironically, although this would be the first year where I could actually qualify as a bona fide member of the squad, I could not play. These kids now have serious slapshots, so Viviën and I watched from the sidelines rather than risk being hit. It was an exciting match. The mums know that the writing is on the wall. In the not too distant future, the kids, with their young legs and their Gretzky hockey camp skills, are going to soundly trounce us, but with a combination of desperation and guile (ending the game early, while one goal up), the mums managed to stave off defeat for one more year. We warmed up around the fire and then sang a bit of "Auld Lang Syne," everyone making up their own version once we pass the well-known first line.

The party is just the thing. Viviën and I are both glad that we're not out on the town in uncomfortable shoes. There seem to be about ten kids, all ages and builds, but they move around so quickly it is difficult to get a head count. There is turkey buffet with all the fixings laid out and a decadent chocolate fountain that runs all night. The fountain is surrounded by platters of fruit, cake, wafers, marshmallows and other things to dip. The endless supply of chocolate keeps the mothers awake and the pack of kids wired until midnight, although at about eleven the kids take on a glassy-eyed flush from all the sugar. I had no idea that little boys could shriek that loudly. Sound waves, in the form of concentric circles actually appear in the glass of cranberry juice I'm holding in response. My friend's little boy has dressed himself in a red tuxedo jacket and top hat covered in glitter. He has taken a fondue stick and made himself a skilful chocolate moustache. He runs around the house trying to kiss everyone's hand and talking in a faux French accent. I love him. And all of these kids are incredibly empathetic and aware of the world around them. Five minutes with these kids, I guarantee, could make just about anyone want a child of their very own. I know because that's exactly what happened to me.

## 67. a prayer upon leaving

After a flurry of activity and a heroic effort in packing and organization on Viviën's part (since I was tied up not only with work but also in doing final rewrites for a play that is debuting in Vancouver), we are ready to head back east. I am feeling remarkably relaxed for someone who is technically homeless and visibly pregnant. Actually, cushy Super 8s and a cozy car will be our temporary home for the next week or so until we make it back to our place in Nova Scotia. We are living the good life.

I am using an internet interface to virtually sit in on the final reading of my play. Last chance to make any more edits that I can hear in the text based on the work the actors are doing. Since our house is all packed up, I am using my small office on the university campus as a home base. While this very important rehearsal transpires it is also the end of term. I try to present a reasonably composed face to the small camera of my laptop, which will show up in the rehearsal hall in Vancouver, while students knock on my door and the baby thrashes around inside me like a spawning salmon.

Since our stuff is going into storage we are getting rid of some of the big pieces that we don't need. This means that for the last few days of packing and getting ready to go, periodically the doorbell rings and folks come in, give us a little stack of cash and haul pieces of furniture away. The house is getting barer and barer. It begins to resemble the abode of the Lou Whos post-Grinch. By now there is almost nothing to sit on, and so when those rare moments occur when we actually have time to sit down and rest, we are using camper recliners. (A camping chair is no joke when you are pregnant.) I've packed so many times that the mere sight of bubble wrap and packing tape, all on their own, can produce in me a frothy cocktail of melancholic nostalgia and irrational rage.

The doorbell rings on our last night in town and I look out the second-floor window to see two fresh-faced men in their twenties. They must be here for the sofa. I am finishing with the upstairs washroom and think I'll just let Viviën handle this one. After a few moments, I realize that the murmur of voices hasn't died away. Their truck is still outside. Surely it can't take that long. *Just give them a discount and say adios*, I think, stepping onto the landing. It is then that I hear the two young men, each still clutching an end of the sofa, trying to convince Viviën to accept Jesus as her personal saviour. Barring that, they are asking for permission to say a prayer over her obviously pregnant belly. Viviën, I can see, is slightly annoyed but still good humoured. She has a light sheen of sweat on her forehead from the packing and has been in the throes of second trimester heartburn all day. Likely she's not in the mood for spiritual guidance, but I know she can handle herself. I keep on packing and hear her telling them that she thanks them for buying our sofa and wishes them well, but that praying and laying on of hands are against house rules.

There are two of them, however, and only one of her. They are speaking in English, and although Viviën's English is impeccable, it is, after all her third language. They are not shrill, they are not offensive, but they are persistent. She needs reinforcements. I'll fast forward through the details because, in structure, any debate between believers and non-believers ends in a tie. Human beings rarely change one another's minds.

The conversation proceeds in a reasonable tone, and we make our way toward agreeing to disagree, but it becomes quickly apparent that the younger of the two is in real distress. He is gesticulating, and I can see a pulsing vein in his neck. This might be because I have now come down the stairs and it is evident that we are both pregnant. Viviën has already mentioned that we are driving back east together, and now the young man blurts out: "I had a vision two days ago and I didn't understand it at the time. The Lord spoke to me and told me I would soon meet two pregnant women journeying east.

"A vision?" I ask, looking toward his friend, who is still holding on to one end of our couch.

"He has visions. He's a prophet. Ask anyone in our congregation," the other young man insists, nodding vigorously. "He's always right on the money. You better let him say his prayer."

Although I am not religious, I have enough superstitious Maritimer in me that the hair on the back of my neck stands up at this moment. We are going to be travelling some very treacherous stretches of road. The Trans-Canada is 8000 kilometres long, tip to tail, much of it scenic, some of it snow covered and passable with caution, and some of it a single-lane death trap. While I have driven it many times from Pacific to Atlantic, I have never done this with a baby on board and a pregnant wife in the dead of winter. Now, we have not only the responsibility of getting ourselves there safely but also our precious cargo.

While the young preacher hasn't managed to strike the fear of god into my agnostic heart, he has successfully freaked me out. He hasn't even blinked an eye about our double-mum family structure and seems genuinely concerned about our well-being. Even if we're not going to drink his Kool-Aid, he is still desperately sure that if we let him say a prayer for us, then we'll make it safely to our destination.

He is so convinced of what he has seen and so earnest that he becomes compelling. We strike a compromise. He says his prayer, and when he reaches for them, we even each give him one of our hands. Viviën and I grow quiet for a moment, each holding one hand of this young stranger as he bows his head. The content of his prayer contains only a wish for our safe travel and well-being. We listen respectfully until he is finished and remain quiet until he raises his head. Regardless of its origin, the benevolence of a stranger is a powerful thing. As he leaves I slip him my copy of *The God Delusion*, a brick of book that, since I've finished reading it (and it isn't the sort you read again for nuance), I need to pass on anyway. To my surprise the young man doesn't take this amiss. He sticks the controversial Dawkins tome under his arm, nods and disappears into the night.

## 68. mamaburger

The trip is going even more smoothly than we dared expect, with clear roads and sunshine every day. We're securing fairly agreeable roadside hotels that have decently comfortable beds and get our rest. We are both fit to drive and feeling good. We are avoiding fast food and instead make pit stops at grocery stores to compose our own hasty but healthy meals. We both still fit behind the wheel (although I am tight at this point), and so we are able to switch drivers every couple of hours and put in respectable days of driving, doing anywhere from six to eight hours, depending on how we feel.

When we first mentioned our plan to drive across the country double pregnant to friends and loved ones, we got some blow-back. What if I go into labour five hours from the nearest hospital and have to deliver the baby in the wilderness? How will Viviën help me, being pregnant herself? What if Viviën goes into labour prematurely? What if — and this probably stretches the laws of probability — we both go into labour at the same time?

Many of these questions that concerned friends and loved ones posed, we had already considered, but it still seemed like our best course of action. Some quantum physicists argue that lingering upon negative possibilities can actually impact the course of events, actually call them into being. The same holds true for positive possibilities, so we're trying to stick with those.

For the most part this strategy is turning out to be pretty effective. We've sailed through a good portion of the trip until we suddenly find ourselves stranded in minus-thirty-eight temperatures in Marathon, an isolated village in Northern Ontario. There has been a bad accident on the only artery connecting the east to the west: a truck from a local mining company collided with a passenger vehicle and then slid across both lanes of the highway. The police holding up traffic tell us that the blockage will be cleared in an hour. No problem. We'll head into town and grab a bite. The only problem is that the town appears to be devoid of anything except a tiny strip mall, an A&W and a very dodgy looking bar. The local people, when pressed, offer that it is theoretically possible to get warm food at the bar — wings and nachos — but they don't remember the last time anyone ordered them and can't vouch for whether they'd be edible. The mere thought of eating nachos, any kind of nachos, let alone stale ones, makes me want to hurl. The problem is that the temperature has now dropped to minus forty. The vomit would freeze mid-air and come back and hit me in the eye. That even more disgusting thought, in turn, makes me want to throw up. I am caught in a morning sickness feedback loop that these days seems to only slow down a bit around 3 p.m., then picks up speed again in the evening.

We head back out to the highway, figuring we'll just wait for the all-clear, then hit the road to the next town. The policeman says again that he expects the blockage to be cleared within the hour. Great. We have to keep the car engine running, of course, to avoid freezing. We listen to the only radio station that has reception as they are providing the most up-to-the-minute news about the blockage. There's a truck in the road, the announcer helpfully informs us, then says he's going to treat us to ten songs in a row before the next update. The station plays all country and western all the time. It must be called WIFELEFT, DOGRANAWAY 101, I joke to Viviën, and this might be funny if we weren't stuck with absolutely nothing else to listen to. The DJ treats us to various remixes of "Achy Breaky Heart" and "Save a Horse, Ride a Cowboy." We try not to watch the red numbers on the car's digital clock as time stretches out, seemingly to infinity. Eventually, we can't help ourselves, we drive up and ask the policeman again how long it will be. He replies again, stony-faced, that the blockage will be cleared within the hour. The problem is that he (or clones of him, they must be switching each other off to avoid freezing to death) stick to this tantalizing story for the entire day and much of the night. We drive to town and back a total of eight times and begin to feel like we're caught in the really cold version of the movie *Groundhog Day*, where the characters are doomed to forever relive the mundane events of the same day. The policeman, now petrified into a flinty caricature of himself, sticks to his story that the blockage will be cleared in an hour.

"But you said that last time, and that was hours ago!" I howl. "And the time before that and the time before that, it's not fair!" The lack of food and the exhaustion are getting to me at this point.

"Ma'am, I am only passing on the information I have," he mouths from behind his frost-encrusted moustache. Finally, we give up and go to the A&W. I waddle up to the counter and try to ironically order a couple of Mama Burgers, but fast foot décor must contain a substance that repels irony. The girl behind the counter is twenty and has died blonde hair with two inches of dark roots. She is visibly excited by the road-blocking accident. In between taking orders, she reports what she knows and pumps customers for new information with an irritating breathlessness. *Is anyone dead? Did they use the jaws of life? Is there at least some blood?* I want to smack her when I go up to get our burgers, but I recognize that this isn't an appropriate course of action. The accident must be the most exciting thing to happen all year up here and she's just a kid. Maybe she's never lost anyone, never been in a car accident herself. I keep scrolling a mental list of excuses for her while jabbing the tips of cold fries in ketchup and trying to force them down.

While the hard orange-and-brown plastic furniture at the A&W certainly wasn't designed with the pregnant woman in mind, the interior of the restaurant does have the obvious advantage of having an ambient temperature above zero. We can only stay in here for a while, however, as the dog is in the car. He'll be okay for forty-five minutes, but after that we'll have to go out and start the engine and heaters again. We realize that we've burned half a tank of gas idling and there is only one gas station in town. What if it has a closing time? We had better head over there and fill up.

"This mama can't eat this Mama Burger," I say.

"Neither can this mama. It's disgusting," Vivïen replies and we tip the rest of what regretfully passed for dinner into the bin and head back out to the car. After another torturous hour or two, we are back on the road. It is 3 a.m. before we make it to the motel we had pre-booked along the road, and we stretch out gratefully on the bed. It will be nice to have the frozen rock of Northern Ontario in the rearview mirror.

## 69. *not Hollywood*

We arrive in Nova Scotia with no further complications and make an appointment at the hospital on the South Shore where we will give birth. They need to do a series of tests in order to begin monitoring both us and the babies. Because this is a whole new world for us, we decide to take the optional tour that is run for couples expecting their first child. The head nurse shows us around the facility. We tour an observation room, a birthing room and a recovery room while she talks us through some possible scenarios of how our birth experience could run.

We are taking this tour with four other couples, and as we enter the birthing room, the nurse indicates some stools and chairs where we are to sit while she answers any questions we might have. Large padded chairs are grouped in pairs with utilitarian wooden stools. The nurse, indicating our swollen bellies, says she's pretty sure the pregnant women need the comfortable chairs. The fathers-to-be head for the stools. The problem comes when we head for our set of chairs. Vivïen is definitely showing and obviously pregnant but is still trying to be tough. She says she's fine with a stool. She's only six months pregnant, after all. She waves me toward the comfy chair. One of the fathers-to-be jumps up and darts into the corridor. He comes back with a padded chair and puts it in the place of Vivïen's stool. It is a little gesture, yet one that goes a great distance toward making us feel at home.

I give him a smile as Vivïen settles in, and the nurse begins talking us through what to expect when we come in to have our babies. She explains that we should come to the hospital either when our water breaks or our contractions are five minutes apart. Then we will be put on the monitor for observation. Every woman's labour is different, she stresses, and the hospital tries hard to accommodate different kinds of births. There are cots available that can be wheeled into the room so that our partner can stay over during the birth process. When we are determined to be in active labour, we will be given a birthing room, but we are free to walk the halls, take a bath, use the birthing ball or the mats and do whatever our bodies tell us. This hospital appears to be remarkably forward thinking compared to some that I read about.

The nurse handles a few more practical questions before she gets to the juicy part: pain relief. I can feel all the pregnant women around the circle shift forward in their chairs. No matter what our views on this subject might be, no matter what kind of birth we hope to have, we all want to hear what she has to say next. The nurse says there are methods of pain relief that work independently and also in conjunction with one another to assist women during the process. Of course breathing, relaxation, movement and bathing are all helpful. If those methods aren't enough, you can request an intramuscular injection of a painkiller such as diamorphine or pethidine, but this must be given early in the labour. If it is too close to delivery, it might slow down the baby's breathing. During the first stages of labour they use a numerical scale to notate the dilation of the uterus. In preparation for birth a woman must go from zero to ten, ten being fully dilated. This process, says the nurse, can be quite painful for some women, while others might only feel a kind of pressure. Once you are in labour, you can request a mask that is connected to a tank of nitrous oxide and oxygen. When you breathe in this gas, it can reduce pain but can also make you feel light-headed and sometimes nauseous. She hauls out the tank and mask to show us what it looks like.

I glance sideways at Viviën to gage her thoughts at this point and notice that she looks woozy. She has low blood pressure, and sometimes if she is ill, or distressed, or even if she sees blood or a needle, she faints. I recognize the twirling dark look in her pupils and lean over to ask her if she is okay.

"Of course the heaviest form of pain relief is the epidural. This is a needle in the back ..." Suddenly the nurse jumps forward in alarm. Just as I am whispering in Viviën's ear, she faints and is sliding down in her chair. Myself and another pregnant woman grab her elbows and help her slide safely to the floor. She has told me this is a terrifying experience for her — she hates the feeling of losing control of her body. So, after helping her to the floor, I talk to her, stroking her back and then her cheek for a few moments until she starts to come around again. My only concern is that Viviën gets through the spell as calmly as possible. But the fathers-to-be, the other pregnant women and even the nurse are all pale with shock. One of the guys offers up his coat as a pillow for her head.

"Well I guess that concludes our tour," the nurse says, shaking her head. "That's the first time I've ever lost one this early in the game."

It gives me a stab of panic to see Viviën's strong body go down this way. Especially when I feel so vulnerable myself. There have only been a couple times when I've questioned the wisdom of what we've done, never the pregnancies themselves, but the timing. Maybe we shouldn't have tried to get pregnant at the same time. Maybe I should have just supported her through this. Am I an idiot? What if I can't get her to the hospital? Doesn't the husband have to drive at Mach 2 through a blinding snowstorm to get his beloved wife to the hospital? Carry her into the emergency room in his arms in the nick of time ... Wait, that's Hollywood.

The unfortunate thing about living in an age so saturated with cinematic images is that they can frequently pull a bait-and-switch on you for the circumstances of your real life. We aren't the Hollywood version of a family. I couldn't carry my woman over the threshold like the hero of the story even if we weren't both pregnant! But just like anyone in love, I would do anything, I mean anything, in the world for her. Whatever we have to do for each other, we've always found the strength for, and this won't be any different.

## 70. nipple stimulation, spicy food & pineapples

The baby is overdue and getting bigger every day. Last night I started comparing percentiles. At the last ultrasound, our son was in the 89th percentile, the kindly nurse told me. Robust. Healthy. Great, that is great,

I am thinking. But I am also remembering that handy and terrifying diagram of cervical openings with what looks like an impossible progression to ten. I am wondering whether my own cervical opening could possibly be in the 89th percentile as well. Somehow I doubt it, so I can't help but busy myself with that maddening physics puzzle.

Tears are, lots of women assure me, normal. Not tears as in crying, although those are likely as well, but tears as in rips. Not words you ever want to associate with your own body, particularly the tender parts. When I ask the doctors and nurses about this, they admit that tears in the perineum — the area between the vagina and the anus — are common. No one likes to think about it, but in fact they are more the rule than the exception. In some cases, an episiotomy is necessary.

"What is an episiotomy?" I ask, already wincing at the sharp edges of the word.

"It is a cut in the perineum that enlarges the opening to allow the baby to be born. These aren't usually necessary unless it is a first pregnancy and the baby is unusually large." That's me, I think. Apparently, research suggests that tears are less severe if they are allowed to occur naturally, without the cut. Although I am eager for more information about this procedure (mostly how to avoid it if possible) and ask a flurry of questions, the doctors only assure me that it isn't life threatening. The nurses are empathetic but are of the opinion that if you can't change something, why dwell on it.

That is an admirable and practical approach, but I can't adopt it and so I read: "First degree tears usually heal on their own. Second and third degree tears affect several pelvic floor muscles that need to be stitched closed, layer by layer." *What!?* Utterly terrified, I read on. "A fourth-degree tear goes through the anal sphincter, causes considerable pain for many months, and increases your risk of anal incontinence." Suddenly I snap the file closed. Perhaps those nurses are right. Best not to dwell on things you can't change. I think I've read enough.

As I've noticed before, the more alarming are the things that happen to your body when you're pregnant, the more everyone assures you that they are normal. This becomes quite maddening after a while. This tearing business does not seem to be normal to me at all. It seems to be some kind of mistake or cruel joke. This whole process is perhaps the only scrap of compelling evidence against a hypothetical supreme being/

creator being female, because it seems doubtful that a woman would set things up this way for herself.

I would really like to start the process, but the baby is showing no signs of ever emerging. He is already a welterweight and gaining by the day. The size differential is only going to get worse, I fear. I wonder aloud whether I might have forgotten to count a few years along the way. If I were forty, a whole different protocol would kick in, and in fact they would not let the baby be overdue at all, they would initiate the birth process artificially. Hey, I start to joke, maybe I am forty really, so perhaps they should help me and out and "induce me," however that is done. The nurse listens to my concerns and says there is a voluntary process that some women insist on having done once they are past their due date. It is called "having your membranes stripped," and it is said to induce labour. She says I should ask the doctor about it.

The doc's answer is less than encouraging. Having your membranes stripped means that the doctor simply dons a rubber glove and plunges her hand up inside you as far as possible. The idea, she explains, is to irritate the cervix, hopefully to the point where it becomes angry enough to react. But this sounds terrible. Why would you want to enrage the very part of your body from which you will need a great deal of cooperation in the near future?

She says briskly that it usually causes a fair amount of bleeding and is quite painful. There isn't a lot of scientific evidence that it actually starts labour, but a lot of women swear by it nonetheless, and she is quite happy to perform it for me if I would like her to.

"Um, I'll pass, thanks. Is there anything else I can do?"

"Yes," she smiles. "You can sit back, relax and wait." And she is out the door to her next patient.

Another nurse has come back inside to check the readings on the baby monitor. She looks at the jagged lines etched on the paper that records the baby's heart rate and movements. She follows the lines down the long scroll of paper, nodding with approval. "Baby doing great," she says. She is wearing whimsical purple scrubs with little green grinning lizards all over them. The way she moves through the space conveys absolute competence, and this in and of itself is balm for our quivering nerves. She has overheard the advice of the doctor, and she has a suggestion of her own. To our surprise, she grabs one of her own nipples and gives it a spritely twist. "Nipple stimulation," she suggests and, with a wink at Viviën, she adds "and lots of sex." During the course of my pregnancy, I have learned that nurses are a breed apart. By necessity, they have none of that squeamishness about the body that plagues mainstream culture. Her job completed, she gives a winning smile to Viviën and whips out the door.

When we arrive back home that evening I consult the internet and come up with a list of things that are supposed to bring on labour: spicy food, sex and pineapples. I'm willing to try all three, but not necessarily in that order. Pineapples are quite prickly.

## 71. from a distance, a penguin

Our first baby is officially five days overdue. He weighs more than many a healthy two-month-old. We have repeatedly requested that the little one make his way to the exit in a timely fashion. The skin across my belly is stretched to the pitch of a conga drum. I am uncomfortable while sitting, standing and lying down. Walking isn't great either. Crouching in public is frowned upon and frequently misread as a social cue. So I am staying at home and reading that trio of insanely popular and lavishly violent Swedish crime novels.

A dirigible, a blimp, a zeppelin … any variety of overinflated vessel could be deployed as a description of the being formerly recognizable as myself. I am slathering on vitamin E and bio oil, hoping against hope that everything will go back into a recognizable shape again after the little guy comes out.

Everything hurts. The baby's kicking and punching my internal organs as if he's training for the infant kick-boxing championship. I haven't given up walking the dog as I am hoping that staying active will precipitate some contractions. At any rate, sitting down and calmly waiting probably won't help. In my black winter coat that won't button up over my white sweatshirt, I must evoke, from a distance, a penguin crossing an ice flow in the Antarctic, which is precisely what our little corner of Nova Scotia looks like right now. Spring? What spring? I failed to consult the *Farmers' Almanac* before planning this birth trip. It says something typical of the crusty charm that I appreciate from the publication. Under weather for eastern Canada, spring 2011, it says: Look Out, White Out!

## 72. letters to possible creatures (on people I wish you'd known)

*There are people with such wonderful smiles in their eyes that their lips don't even have to move to make you feel warm and safe. Your great grandmother was one of these. I wish you could have visited her in her white with green trim house high above the ocean with its windblown apple trees and tall maples and sit with her on the corner of the artisan well and see if you could hear the apples growing. I wish you could play in the back field where old cars are put out to pasture when they stop running and the lupines grow up over their bumpers in a wash of white, pink and purple. I wish you could spend time at her elbow, peering over the edge of the worn kitchen table and learn how to really beat the pants off someone in a game of Chinese checkers. I wish you could smell her baked beans sweet with molasses.*

*It makes me very sad sometimes when I think that you'll never get to meet her yourself. All you'll have are stories from me, and a few pictures, to give you an idea. But then I think that, in a way, you are her. Or a little bit of her anyway. Maybe you'll get her long toes like I did. Maybe you'll get her laugh or her smile.*

*When you lose someone you can't bear to lose, there is a trick you can use. You can imagine that you have their eyes and that you carry them around inside of you so that everything you see, everywhere you go, every beautiful sight, like the blue of the water off a Greek island, the whorl of smooth pink inside a conch shell or the amazing pattern in the bark of one of the oldest trees on earth ... as you see it, they can see it somehow through your eyes and in this way they can share it with you.*

## 73. *following survivor*

The hospital is a world unto itself. From the inside, everything that happens makes perfect sense and operates with a clicking whirring logic all its own. Time takes on a speed that outsiders will never understand. The personages are larger than life. The doctors and nurses literally hold life and death in their hands every single day. And for the most part they still find time to make eye contact and ask you how you're feeling.

Everything inside this self-contained world is heightened and extreme. You might pass a man in the hallway who has just lost his beloved. You might walk by a woman who just brought her firstborn into the world. Joy, agony — it is not a place for nuance. It is not a place of contemplation, but one of rest and sudden action. You look into the nurse's room and you seem to see three or four women gossiping, nibbling graham crackers and watching TV, but all it takes is a *code blue* over the PA and those same women transform into an awesome swat team, springing into action to kick the butt of pain and suffering.

When you arrive for the first time on the maternity ward, the nurses know, especially if it is your first child, that you'll likely be a repeat customer. You'll beat a path between your home and the monitoring room for a week, maybe more, before it's really show time. *Get comfortable* is their mantra. They teach you how to attach the monitor to your belly. They explain what the etched lines on the readout mean and how to adjust the sticky cups if they fall off. Viviën and I make a bit of a splash in the maternity ward. When we go in for check-ups, all the nurses come over to meet and say hello to the hospital's first double pregnant lesbian couple.

As it turns out we have lots of time to get to know everyone. Our first son has no intention of showing up on time. Between all the visits scheduled for Viviën, who is seven months pregnant, and for me, at term, we are near daily visitors. I know what the head nurse takes in her coffee. We've heard the life stories of many of the other nurses as we sit, hour by hour, with a beeping monitor on one or other of our bellies. Heart rates and activity levels are monitored. Many popsicles are eaten. The frozen sugar water passes through the blood to the babies and gets their activity levels going.

"I am seeing red spots and tiny twinkly points of light," I tell one of the nurses, when I am a few days overdue. I am hoping she'll say that this is the first sign of a quick and painless delivery.

"Yes, that can happen. Here stick this on your belly," she says. "Are you following *Survivor* this season?"

"Following *Survivor*?" I say. "This baby is going on two weeks overdue and he's nearly ten pounds, I think I'm living it!"

"There, there," the nurse says, chuckling. She is probably a few years younger than me, but in this situation she is the wise authority and I am the greenhorn. She actually pats my head. It is affectionate, not condescending, and she seems so relaxed that I can feel my own tension dropping. She offers me the other half of a purple popsicle, which I pop into my mouth and suck in sullen silence.

## 74. we have created enchantment

The baby is now close to three weeks overdue, and I've had nothing more than butterflies in my tummy. The tension is literally and figuratively unbearable. I can't really stand up straight or get up off the floor. This is of course (what else) completely normal, the nurses assure me when I get to the hospital. After consulting a chart, the nurse tells me they'll be able to induce me today. What this means is that they'll insert a tubule of prostaglandin gel, which will soften and thin out the cervix in preparation for labour and hopefully also start some contractions.

The insertion of the gel is no more uncomfortable than the cervical exam, which by now I am accustomed to. The only difference is that this time, afterward, it feels as if I have inadvertently gotten some hot sauce down there. It isn't painful exactly, but I definitely feel something. After the insertion, it is back on the monitor. They check the baby and ensure that he is doing fine, but I am still not having any measurable contractions. A few moments later, I go to the washroom and discover that I've passed a blood clot the size of a hot dog bun. Alarmed, I tell this to the nurse.

"Excellent! You're doing great," she says. "You know you all don't have to hang around here, you can go out and walk around the mall if you like. There are some really cute baby jumpers on special at Zellers."

"Thank you," I say. But I am thinking: *Are you for real? I'm not going to Zellers, I could bleed to death! I could drop the baby in aisle five. I'm staying right here, thanks.* We go out into the waiting room, which is specifically for the maternity section of the hospital. A coven of grandmothers sits near the door, relishing the drama vicariously.

"How many centimetres are you?" one of them calls out, by way of greeting. They have been around this horn before and don't give a hoot what is overheard by the cluster of fathers and grandfathers gathered around some fuzzy sports on a TV in the corner.

"Not far, two or three. I just had the gel." Ah, the gel, yes the gel, they nod. "Not doing much yet, just feels like hot sauce!" I quip and the ladies all laugh.

The next time they bring me in for an exam, the obstetrician is there, and she decides that enough is enough. "We are going to help you out here. I'm going to break your water, okay?" she asks briskly and I nod. Before I even have time to think about it, I feel a short sharp poke. This is followed by a flood of hot salty amniotic fluid. There is so much of it, it soaks my clothes and the bed and gushes onto the floor. Even the nurses and doctor, who no doubt are used to this kind of thing, take a step back to avoid the splash. Before I know what is happening, two people are lifting me up and another is scooting out all of the soaked material underneath. I am glad that things are finally in motion after all the waiting. I can even feel some of the tension go out of the overstretched drum of my belly. This semi-relaxation lasts for about four and a half minutes as they move me over to the birthing room, and then wham. Something hits me from a source I can't locate. It's like being sucker punched in the abdomen by the invisible man. I lose control of my muscles and buckle in half like a jackknife. *Oh, that must be a contraction,* I think to myself, *initiate calm, controlled deep breathing sequence.* In a matter of seconds, however, another one hits and stronger. This one is in my back and side. The nurse on duty looks up from her chart with surprise.

"That's a bit close together." She tells me to watch the clock and says that I should get a bit of relief between contractions, but this doesn't happen. They just come one on the back of the other with no pause in between.

What happens next is, for the first time, not entirely normal. I catapult into full-on labour even though I am nowhere near where I need to be on the dilation scale in order to deliver the baby. They call the head nurse, who is a model of efficiency. She begins asking me questions, but by now I can't speak. I am so afraid there is something wrong, so afraid for the baby. I am collapsed against her shoulder, my face a running mess of mucus as she speaks into my ear. Hands hold a gas mask out to me, and they show me how to take a breath and then take it away from my face when I exhale. The mask amplifies the sound of my own gasping.

The anesthesiologist takes a long time to arrive. When he gets here, he has, of course, a protocol to follow. A clipboard is put under my nose, but it becomes apparent that in my animal state I will be of no use with a pen. Viviën reads and signs on my behalf. The next thing I hear is a man saying they will have to hold me down.

"If she move, I maybe lose needle in her back. She could be paralyze," he says in his antiseptic eastern European accent. This phrase is about the strongest motivator a person could have for holding stock still, and I fasten myself onto the bedrail with everything I've got. I am a block of stone, I say to myself, but the jack-knifing motion doesn't seem to be in my control. He has to hurry. Another one is coming. Another one is coming for me. They put a towel in my mouth. I bite it. Or is it a towel? I am biting on something, maybe it is a gas mask? I am terrified and even more so because I can see Viviën's face contorted in fear. What if this sends her into early labour, or what if it hurts our other baby, I think to myself and feel an extra stab of panic. I don't have control of anything physical or emotional. I am nothing more than a twisting double helix of pain. The head nurse has me in some kind of half nelson trying to keep me flat as the contractions hit.

"This is the anesthesiologist," she says. "He is now going to put a needle in your back, and then the pain will go away, but you have to be very still.

"Tighter," I manage to squeeze out between clenched teeth. "Hold me tighter."

When pain hits a certain point, it takes on a texture and a life force of its own. I feel a separation as if I am rising up out of my body, but it only lasts for a second or two, until a contraction hits and pulls me back to earth like a chain about my ankle. I don't want anyone else near me except this near stranger who I passed once in the hallway today and she nodded a welcome. I am soaking the front of her shirt with my tears, and

I can feel her stroking the back of my head, telling me I am going to be okay. I want to believe her.

Time passes, I am not sure how much, and gradually as the medication takes the edge off the pain it feels like I can pull up to the surface and take a breath. My mother and my aunt come in and out, asking if I need anything and making sure I am okay. I close my eyes for a moment, and when I open them I am alone. There is a different nurse now, who looks up from the book she is reading and asks if I need anything.

"The baby is fine. Your wife is resting in the next room. You just rest too and let your body catch up to where you are supposed to be."

We pass a few more hours of the night in this way. She with her book and me drifting between sleep and waking. Every so often the baby warming machine fires up with a whoosh. It needs to stay at a certain temperature so it periodically turns on with clicks and whirs. The first couple of times it is frightening, but by now I consider it an ally. It will catch the baby in his first few moments of life on the outside. It will take his vital signs and keep him at a perfect temperature as he takes his first breaths.

It's not over yet. It's not sleep that I'm in. It's not awake either. It's somewhere in the middle, some kind of somnolent pre-pouncing state, my body gathering strength beneath me. The nurse tells me to relax and let my body do the work for me now. Just let your mind go, she says. For now, just let everything go.

The pain never really goes away, and I can feel it hunting me through the barricades. Toward morning the medication is stopped, and the pain begins to gain on me again. The doctor comes in to check and then tells me that it is fine, I am dilated properly and can now give birth. It is okay if the feeling comes back now, he says, you need to feel the urgency to a certain degree in order to push.

Suddenly I find a wall of muscle that I didn't know existed. In my head I see flashes of choppy light, as if the light is being hacked into bits by a ceiling fan. Flashes of light on stone. *I can't do thi*s, I think. Then *I have to do this.* Just bright sunlight on stone. Now it's a form.

"The baby needs to come out now," one of the nurses says. "He needs air."

I squint my eyes and try to make out the form under my eyelids. I can hear encouraging noises from the room but not words any more.

A spasm and I feel my back arch as if electricity is passing through me. I know Viviën is there, she is holding my hand, and her grip is keeping me tethered to earth. I can see the form now. It's Atlas, the Titan, stone muscles hoisting the world aloft. Finally something gives. Everyone cheers. There are only three or four people in the room, but to my ears it sounds like a crowd bursting into applause blended with the outraged cry of the baby as he takes his first shocking breath. There he is, they hold him up and I reach for him, but he has to go to the warming machine for a moment. They check him over. Can't find a thing wrong with him, the doctor jokes, and then they lay him on my chest. His blue eyes slide open and peer into mine. He is here, he is beautiful.

"We made it," I say to Viviën. "Only one more to go."

I take one look back over my shoulder. It is as if there is a blasted bridge, burned wreckage behind us, but now we're in the clear. I want to get up out of the bed and take him home right now.

"Let's go home," I say and start to get up.

"No," they say, "you have to stay here for a bit. You have to deliver the afterbirth, and the doctor needs to do a repair on you."

"A repair?"

"You need stitches. You have a tear and the doctor needs to stitch you up."

*Can't think about that. He's here. We made it.* His feet are blue, which is normal they tell me, and I am relieved to hear this word again. They are already starting to pink up even as we speak. We name him as his eyes open toward us. They are a deep rich blue and seem already to be taking us in.

I hear Blanche Dubois's voice whispering deep into my ear: *Oh look, she says, we have created enchantment.*


## 75. sleep of the righteously exhausted

It is in the wee hours of the next night and I am awake. The danger has passed, and our new baby son is sleeping peacefully in the crook of Viviën's arm. He is nestled against the warm mass of his little brother still snug in Viviën's belly. I don't know how she has done this at seven months pregnant, but she has found the strength to clean our son and rock him to sleep, and now they are both deep in the sleep of the righteously exhausted. I can see tiny, ever so slight stirrings in her taut belly where our second baby floats comfortably in his liquid world, with no idea about the journey that lies ahead for him. I try to turn over and feel a hard, painful rock on my chest. It is my own breast that has suddenly, violently filled with milk. I struggle to get up in a tangle of sheets, an IV line and the pool of my own blood that I am lying in. At this moment, it doesn't seem as if I'll ever be able to get up, get clean and heal. I feel as if I am too wrecked to ever be myself again.

All through the day adrenaline kept us going as family, friends and even strangers came in, one after the other, to look at our new arrival. Most of these visits were lovely, everyone oohing and ahhing along with us and taking delight in our newly arrived son. The visits of some women though, especially older women, had a bizarre edge. They relentlessly pursued details regarding the birth and then uniformly told us to count our lucky stars. They themselves, or their daughter, daughter-in-law, niece, etc., they assure you, had it much worse.

"Consider yourself lucky, I dropped my baby in the hallway," said one. "We were waiting for a bed, I was screaming, leaning against the railing and my husband went to beg for a doctor. Nobody believed me that I was going to have her and then wham, out she came: right on the floor of the hallway. Then they came running with a gurney. A little late, aren't ya, I said."

We were regaled with tales of babies born on the side of the highway. Babies that came out entirely blue and had to be resuscitated, mothers who had to take two months' bed rest after giving birth, you name it. I wondered at the quality of these stories. The tellers seemed almost to revel in the violence and danger, to savour their closeness to matters of life and death. The mothers-in-law in particular had a concealed knife blade in their words. Something in the storytelling resembled the way that soldiers tell others war stories, their brushes with death in battle. And I guess that makes utter sense.

One woman, whose daughter-in-law was still in labour, came into our room. She'd heard somehow that I had a tear during delivery, and she hovered, buzzardlike, at the foot of my bed. "My daughter-in-law had such bad tearing with her first one that afterward what she had down there didn't even look like a vagina."

*Dear god. Don't you have some place you should be.*

"It'll make delivering the next one easier, they say. But all she's got down there is just two big flaps, like curtains, hanging any old way …" I held my hand up to her, as if I could form a physical barrier between myself and her words, and waved my other hand to my loved ones. *Please, please, can someone get her out of here?*

All of this goes through my mind as I lie here in the silence of the ward. I desperately want to get up and to clean myself, but I can't. And I don't want to disturb those three beings all resting there on the fold-out cot. I manage to soundlessly wave down a nurse as she passes in the hallway. She puts a finger to her lips, nodding, and helps me to the bathroom without waking everyone. She has an accent that I recognize. First, I think it is from Newfoundland, with the lilting musicality and the foreshortened vowels, but she says she hails from Cape Breton. Her steady compassion is the remedy for my dark thoughts. She helps me disentangle, making small soothing noises in her throat.

"Had a rough go of it, haven't you, my love." She jokes about the indignity of the grannie panties I'm wearing — huge ungainly disposable underwear with large pads to soak up the blood. I am alarmed by my swollen breasts, and she checks them and (no surprise) tells me they are normal. "First time your milk comes down, it comes with a vengeance," she says, smiling. "Better than a boob job." Not for the first time I think you have to be gifted with a very special combination of personality and skills to do this job well, and even in my miserable state, I admire her. Before long she has me cleaned up and back in bed, and I, too, find the sleep of the righteously exhausted.


## 76. unlearning

I was prepared to abandon myself to this experience, and it's a good thing. I'll begin an email only to find it again, unfinished, three days later. By which point the world will have moved on, not having been thrown off course by the failure of my message to arrive. All of that is quite beside the point, says the baby in a poignant howl. *I need a change. I need to drink. I would like to listen to Bob Marley while being held, cuddled and danced about the room. And now I would like to go over to the window so as to contemplate the angle of the morning light on the Atlantic as the inland fishermen check their lobster traps.* I peer into his eyes … blue as most infant's eyes are in the beginning but with streaks of gray and green. He is right, he'll only be a newborn once. Everything else will keep.

His look is so incredibly serious. Whenever I look into an infant's eyes I can't help wondering if perhaps we aren't born with some secret store-house of knowledge. Given all that we do not know about the brain, isn't it possible that each of us is born knowing everything? What if we arrive on earth knowing the solution to the Hodge conjecture, the method for carving a perfectly formed human skull against the grain from a single quartz crystal, all of the digits of pi and all the rest of the vast ocean of human knowledge? What if instead of learning, we simply unlearn as we grow up? Perhaps slowly, ever so slowly, like stones wearing down into grains of sand on a beach, the edges of this vast intelligence wear away, the edges come off of it to a degree that we can then communicate with one another.

Our son's gaze at the moment seems to contain all imaginable knowl-edge along with a storehouse of punch-lines for excellent jokes and a foolproof plot to overthrow the government. It seems inconceivable that we could recover from something like the birth process at all, let alone in a week. But here we are with our firstborn son as stars wink in the night sky and the lights spill across the becalmed harbour, getting ready to do it all again in a few weeks.


## 77. of zen & concrete

Life, by necessity, has become simple in the extreme. Uncomplicated in its complete devotion to the essential things in life: sleep, nourishment, water, fresh air. Being up until now an unrepentant multi-tasker, a late-night meeter of deadlines, a taker-on of too many projects, this is my first brush with radical simplicity. The minutes and hours slip by as we peer into our son's eyes, wondering whether that smile on his lips is attributable to gas or mirth, trying to gauge his reactions to the fresh salty air, to his first bath, and to the music we play for him. I have never been, really, much of a meditator, and don't think I have a zen bone in my body. At least I didn't, but caring for the baby and also for ourselves in this delicate time seems to bring on this state by necessity. Light, space and even time take on prismatic qualities.

That is until Viviën decides we need to pour concrete. Yes, concrete. Ready-mix cement to be poured into the cardboard moulds that will underpin the small outbuilding we've decided to build down by the water. Even though she is quite close to her due date and could go into labour at any moment, somehow Viviën gets it into her head that we must complete the foundations for the building before she goes into the hospital. Just the foundation, she assures me — she won't frame up the building itself until after she's actually given birth. Well that's a comfort, I think. At first, I try to dissuade her. I don't want her to be lifting things, but she promises that she'll only supervise. Also, I am in a kind of thrall to our firstborn son that I am supposing is a natural state and don't want to be more than a few feet from him at any time. We compromise by bringing him out onto the deck, where he sleeps in his baby seat in the fresh air while I dig the holes in the ground in which to place the concrete moulds.

People in Lockeport have gotten used to us by now, but the sight of a very pregnant woman out in the yard with a cement mixer will still turn a head or two. The fishermen slow down as they drive by on their way to the wharf. *What will they think of next?* they seem to say as they shake their heads and wave.

## 78. on the monitor

I love the utter unconventionality with which Viviën wears her pregnancy. For some bizarre reason it seems as if all women, no matter what their fashion sense or personal style prior to becoming pregnant, go in more and more heavily for floral prints, ruffles and chenille (sometimes nauseatingly combined on one article of clothing) the closer they get to their delivery date. Maybe this is due simply to an oversight on the part of the makers of maternity clothes everywhere. At any rate, Viviën does not go softly into chenille and floral print. She steadfastly refuses to wear maternity clothes, opting only for larger versions of her usual attire, worn in slightly more forgiving ways. As she makes her way back and forth to the maternity ward in her high top basketball sneakers, cap and jeans slung low on her hips, you could mistake her for a visitor riding the elevator up to see a loved one … if it weren't for that gorgeous and outrageous belly.

For the past few days we have been beating the familiar path between our place and the hospital every couple of days as Viviën's due date approaches and then passes. Our second son seems as reluctant as his brother to make his appearance, and Viviën has felt nothing at all in the way of contractions. Maternity protocol in Nova Scotia dictates that because of her age, Viviën should not go more than a week past her due date, and so she is put on the list to be induced.

We expect her to be taken in within the next forty-eight hours to be given the prostaglandin gel and hopefully begin Act II of our great adventure. There is, however, an immediate epidemic of women going into labour the old-fashioned way, and she gets bumped down the list until some beds clear up. They still want to see her once per day and put her on the monitor, so we decide that driving back and forth is too taxing. We camp out in a motel a couple of blocks away from the hospital and wait for her to go into labour or for a spot to come up so that they can induce her. The first day is great. We relax in the motel eating order-in food and watching cable TV — two things that aren't available in our little ocean house. Viviën is feeling good and the baby is sleeping well at night in his little fold-out crib. They try the gel on Viviën, but it doesn't seem to have an effect; she says she doesn't feel anything. She is getting tired of waiting and also tired of the motel. She wants to go back home and sleep in our own bed. I convince her that we should stay close by, as it seems foolhardy to have a newborn baby, a wife in labour and a stretch of long windy single-lane highway between us and the hospital right now. One night stretches into two, three, then four however, as we are continually bumped again by gals going into labour.

We are lucky to have some family members living nearby, and they visit us, bring fruit trays and organize barbeques. We can feel the love and warmth pouring around us on all sides and it is wonderful. If it weren't for the trial that Viviën will still have undergo it could feel like one long vacation.

At the motel in the evenings we watch the basketball finals. On the evening of the fifth day, the hospital finally calls Viviën in and tells her they will try the gel again. They insert the gel and say she'll need to stay on the monitor for an hour. She tells me that I should take the baby back to lie down. She can call me when she is finished or else get a cab back to the hotel. She feels nothing at all and doesn't expect the gel to do anything this time either. I don't want to leave her there, but the baby is getting fussy, so I take him back to our room and wait by the phone. About an hour later, Viviën arrives back. She had a burst of energy and decided to walk. This gives me a lump in my throat.

"Why didn't you call me? What if you went into labour on the side of the road?" I ask.

"I would have flagged someone down," she says. "I just really needed the fresh air, I needed to walk."

We start to watch the game, and no more than five minutes pass before she gets a contraction. A real one. She stretches out on the bed and rides it out. Then she gets another, but there are still fairly big gaps between them. We time them because they have told us at the hospital that there is no use in coming there until the contractions are about five minutes apart. Otherwise, you could just end up being on the monitor for an hour, then sent back home again. Viviën would rather try and work up to it gradually, here in comfort. I understand this but also know I'll have to get her and the baby into the car and over to the hospital. I don't want things to progress to the point where I'll no longer be able to do this and have to call an ambulance. This seems silly when we are just down the street. I fetch her drinks and cubes of fresh fruit to build up her strength and try not to pace.

Just after half-time, her labour hits in earnest. We have her things together, and I put our son in the car seat, then go back for Viviën. At this moment I am so thankful that we decided to stay in the motel. Her contractions are hitting closer and closer together, but the hospital is only two blocks away. We pull up to the emergency entrance, drop off Viviën, and then I park the car and unhook the car seat. Our first son, thankfully, is still asleep in the detachable seat and I carry him inside that way. In the lobby a kindly old gentleman looks us over. He looks at Viviën, and then down at our baby asleep in the car seat.

"They don't take 'em back ya know, there's no return policy," he quips, and Viviën manages to smile at this. She is doing great, but I am relieved to have her back in the hands of the nurses. Here we go, I think, and mentally try to prepare myself for the night ahead. Everyone on the maternity ward remembers us. They give us one of their extra newborn incubator cots for our firstborn son to sleep in. He is already such a big baby that he dwarfs the cot.

Whenever anyone sees him, now nearly two months old and very big for his age, they give a start — thinking he is a truly giant newborn. I try to reassure the pregnant women walking the halls and get very good at summing up the story of our little family in ten words or less.

Viviën has everything totally in hand. She is easing into the contractions, breathing deeply and relaxing like a pro. I am so happy there isn't the panic we had the first time around. We settle into a room for the night and have a talk with the nurse who'll be working with us. Based on how things are going she expects Viviën to gradually prepare herself to deliver and perhaps have the baby in the wee hours of the morning. We know all the nurses from our last, very recent trip, and they are tickled by the novelty of the situation. Even with her busy schedule, our nurse has time to cuddle the baby and help me get him down for the night. We have a cot for me, as it seems like we'll be staying here overnight. The contractions come and go. I fetch popsicles and pieces of fruit for Viviën when she needs them. She is in a state that I recognize: concentrated and interior, almost trancelike. Our son, thankfully, is sleeping the night away while his mama gets ready to deliver him a little brother. Sometime in the middle of the night, I pass out on the cot, exhausted.

I wake to the sound of Viviën being sick. I didn't hear her calling so she rang the buzzer. The nurse comes in and checks her and says that Viviën has made it, she's fully dilated.

"Well done!" she says to Viviën. "That's a lot of the hard work done already. I'll call the doc now." She puts in a call to the doctor on duty, and we both take one of Viviën's hands, assuring her it won't be long now. Some relief seems to come to the surface of Viviën's face though she is still far, far away, concentrating on the task at hand. The nurse and I chat a bit, trying to distract Viviën. The nurse puts in another call. "Shouldn't be long now," she says. More time passes. She puts in a third call, and I can see annoyance start to stamp itself on her brow. "Should be here by now," she says. Still the doc does not come.

The nurse says she has no idea what the hold-up could be, but she tells Viviën that we can't wait any more and she can start to push any time. And push she does. The effort, I can see, is amazing. Her strength is amazing. I thought I loved her as much as it was possible for one human being to love another. Watching her labour in this way to bring our baby into the world unlocks a whole set of floodgates I didn't know existed. She grips the rails of the bed and pulls on them until it seems she is bending the metal of the bars.

The nurse and I both coach Viviën. We remind her to breathe, we pass her the mask and drinks of water when she asks for them. About forty-five minutes pass, but there is still no doctor. Viviën labours and labours, and finally here comes the fluid and some blood, and we can just see the very top of the baby's head!

We urge Viviën on, the nurse now preparing everything to deliver the baby herself. She tells me what to do to help her since the doctor hasn't arrived. Then something happens. At the moment when Viviën appears to have reached the apex of her effort, it really feels like the baby should come right out ... he does not. Something changes in Viviën's voice, and it just seems as if something is wrong. The nurse puts in another call this time, very urgent. She tells Viviën to stop pushing. This is the only moment, during all of it, when I hear Viviën let out a cry. Up until now, she had been breathing and vocalizing but all with a measure of control. When they tell her to stop pushing, when everything in her body and mind and soul is telling her to bring that baby out, she starts to cry and the sound is heart wrenching.

Finally, the doc gets here. She is groggy, bleary-eyed. Her manner is super casual, and she is clearly expecting it to be hours before anything of interest will happen. I've observed how medical personal cultivate calm and try to spread it around like a tonic, and in most cases I appreciate this. But right now her casual manner is driving both the nurse and me into fits, and I am most concerned that it might be costly to Viviën and the baby.

I hate to judge people by appearances, but the doc is wearing some old acid-washed t-shirt, fuzzy jogging pants and sneakers that had their best days in 1982. Her hair hangs lank and greasy over her face, and her absentminded manner does nothing to inspire confidence. There is a kind of torpor in her, as if she were one layer back from reality. Maybe she's taken sleeping pills. I don't know what it is, but I can see that our nurse is losing patience with her, and Viviën looks terrified.

The doctor painstakingly gets herself organized to check Viviën. She puts a monitor on the baby's head. The nurse and I, knowing what all the readings mean, watch as the baby's heart rate dips alarmingly.

"I'm just tickling his head," says the doctor. "He doesn't seem to like having his head tickled on that side."

Then his heart rate drops again. The nurse and I lean forward, and the doctor's eyes bug out, but she seems frozen in place. Suddenly she says we need to turn Viviën over — she has to sit up onto her hands and knees and this will instantly get the baby more air. We manage to do this, although Viviën is in a lot of pain. I have no idea where she's finding the strength to stay up on her hands and knees. There are beads of sweat all over her body, she is quivering, shaking, her whole body knotted against the urge to push.

"You need to phone this in," says the nurse to the doctor. When she still doesn't move, the nurse barks: "Now!"

And finally, finally, the doctor makes the call. Within minutes there is a swat team of highly capable doctors and nurses around us. The obstetric surgeon assesses Viviën and lets us know in a few words what has happened. The baby has turned posterior, and in her experience, once a baby turns this way, there is rarely a successful vaginal birth. To continue would be dangerous for the baby and very dangerous for the mother. Her advice is for Viviën to be sedated and have an emergency C section. We agree and she asks me if we are married. I say yes, and she nods, saying, "Great, that makes things easier." I quickly sign the consent forms on Viviën's behalf. I wish that anyone who doesn't agree with gay marriage — based on whatever kind of convictions they have — would have to stand in these shoes for one moment. I wonder how they would feel if they didn't have the power to give consent for their partner. What if precious seconds were lost while the authorities sorted out the red tape and their loved one's life hung in the balance. This is life and death right here, it doesn't get more basic.

In a matter of minutes, the team stabilize the baby and put Viviën into sedation. Everything is going to be fine now, they reassure her and me. We have a monitor on the baby's head. Everything is going to be just fine. Viviën, heroic, exhausted and really at the end of the labour, sinks down onto the mattress. They tell me to get into hospital scrubs so that I can go into the operating room with her. I do this at lightning speed, but when I come back something has shifted, the protocol changed, and I must wait outside. I don't care at this point. I just don't want to take one second of anyone's time who needs to be helping Viviën and the baby.

Our firstborn son, meanwhile, is sleeping through all of this and I am so grateful. I worry that if he wakes and cries he might distract the doctor and the team, but the kind of concentration these people cultivate, I quickly understand, cannot be marred by a crying baby. It is as if he somehow senses that he needs to sleep this one through, and so sleep on he does until the wee hours of the morning, when I call my mother, who comes right over to take care of him.

Not much time at all passes, but to me pacing the hallway in hospital greens a whole lifetime could be going by. Then, through the door, I hear the impossibly loud stereophonic cry of our second son. Inside the delivery room, everyone bursts into applause as if their team has scored, which indeed it has. One of them opens the door a crack so that I can peer inside and see our second son as he emerges whole and beautiful. He is not a large baby but his strength is evident in the way he fills his lungs and makes himself heard throughout the ward. Despite his ordeal, he is entirely hale and healthy other than a huge bump on the side of his head, which is (that word again) normal and will disappear in the next few days. His hands and feet are blue like our firstborn's were. He leans his head back as he puts his whole body into the cry. His mouth is so open wide that it is nearly as big as his whole head, and he shakes his adorable fists and pummels the air in sheer shock at being dumped so rudely into the outside world.

He has to go in an incubator for a short time, just to acclimatize to the temperature, but they hand him to me, wrapped up tight, to hold for a moment. They tell me Viviën will not be awake for quite a while, and so I am to take him to the incubator room. I put my hands inside the incubator and hold him, so that he can feel my touch, and this calms him. For the first time since his birth, inside the warmth of the incubator where I stroke him gently, so gently, he calms down.

As soon as I am allowed to, I take him back to Viviën. They tell me she won't be awake for some time yet, but the first thing I want her to see, when she even begins to wake up, is both of us there and the baby safe and sound. Being put under anesthetic is disorienting, and I don't want her to even have one second of fear for our new baby boy when she wakes. As soon as her eyes begin to focus we are there: me, holding her hand, and our second son swaddled and content in the crook of her arm, his brother waiting for us in the arms of my own mother down the hall.

## 79. a new project

The next time we emerge into the fresh air our little family is complete. Two mums and two beautiful baby boys. Viviën is mending in record time. The incision that brought our second son into the world is a barely visible line on the way to disappearing. The bump on the baby's head is nearly gone, and hour-by-hour he seems more at ease. It is quite a production loading everything and everybody into the car as we leave the hospital, but we have lots of help from my mother, my aunt and one of our favourite nurses. Our dog Rockit is in the car as we pack up and get the car seats in place. His eyes register some disbelief that we are bringing another one of those small noisy people home, but he takes it with good will. We pull out of the parking lot, and the hospital (a world onto itself) fades in the rearview. As I pilot my precious cargo along the ninety minutes of winding shoreline road back to Lockeport, I feel suddenly the weight of responsibility, not just for getting them all home safely, but for taking care of all of them — wife, sons and puppy — to varying degrees for the rest of my life. I feel ready to give it my all every single day.

In our little summer house on the southernmost tip of Nova Scotia on the lip of the Atlantic we have the rest of the year to love, feed, bathe, read to, teach, learn from and play with our babies. We eat fresh seafood and push the stroller along the beach over lumps of seaweed, fresh salty air filling those new little lungs. Life again returns to its most basic: food, water, rest and love. Some evenings when we put them down to sleep, we resort to peanut butter sandwiches for supper, but we eat them together, happily, with our feet up, pleased with what we have accomplished. Just as this zen-like state has returned and the late spring sun bouncing off the water is lulling me into a comfortable routine, Viviën begins staring out the window at the concrete pilings down on the waterline.

"I would like to get started soon" is all she says, and knowing her as I do, I understand that there is really no point in trying to change her mind. In fact, by the end of the afternoon, our plans to put up a little woodshed have escalated into a full-on extra building complete with hardwood and tile interior that will serve as a small guesthouse/office.

And this is how it is that I find myself in the house, breastfeeding one baby and rocking the other to sleep with my foot while Viviën, six weeks to the day from the moment she brought our son into the world, frames up beams for the new building. She has a team of two great guys working with her: my cousin and another hardworking guy with a sunny disposition on a work exchange from the U.K. They know us a little bit by now and don't even blink when I bring our youngest son out for his feeding time.

"The boy would like a word," I say.

"I'm coming. I just want to finish this last beam," says Viviën from the ladder, around a couple nails she has squeezed between her lips. Our son registers his impatience with a hearty howl, waving his two little fists in the air.

"He really won't take no for an answer," I say. She comes down from the ladder, and the fellows laugh as they put down their tools. They come and sit on the step to sip a cold beer and eat the sandwiches I made for them.

No matter how long we live on this planet and how many changes we go through together, I shall always carry this snapshot of Viviën close to my heart: her strong arms cradling our son as she feeds him, the Atlantic a piercing blue behind her, sawdust resting lightly on her hair and arms, and her eyes glinting with the excitement of a new project.

## Acknowledgements

Many thanks to the excellent first readers of this manuscript: Chapelle Jaffe, Kathleen Tudor and Beth Everest. The scope and breadth of your collective intellect inspired me when I sat down with your annotated first drafts. The questions you raised fueled the editing process and enlivened this book beyond measure. I also acknowledge the mentors, colleagues and fellow artists and writers who gave me guidance, encouragement and inspiration for this work: Kate Millet, Aritha Van Herk, Kate Reid, Sara Grafe and Inge Fraters.

Thanks to the members of "Write On," a writers group that meets in the Lockeport library, whose members at the time I attended were Kathleen Tudor, Danielle Williams, Kay Daly, J. MacConnell, Shelby Kelly, Shirley Townsend, Marguerite Herff and Gretchen Markle. As a playwright I usually have the comfortable device of character through which to write what is closest to my heart. To turn the pen on oneself is a frightening prospect. You heard the early raw drafts of this book, and your laughter, support and encouragement were invaluable.

Many thanks to Beverley Rach and everyone at Roseway. Also to Brenda Conroy for your keen editor's eyes, gentle humour and attention to detail.

A big thank you to Glenda Stirling, the folks Lunchbox Theatre, director Pamela Halstead and the cast of the first reading of *Speed Dating for Sperm Donors*. This stage play, a fictionalized version of some of the events that take place in the book, is a full-on, knee-slapping comedy about sperm donation that I was working on at the same time as this book. I doubt I would have gone for it whole hog without your support and encouragement.

We are so grateful to friends and family in Holland and Canada, who encouraged and supported us during the time we were trying to have babies ... and then reached out with open arms to hold them as soon as they arrived.

Finally, we are profoundly grateful to every man who came out to meet us, ate a dinner or shared a coffee or a walk in the park and who took time out of his day to come and explore the prospect of helping us have a baby.